DON'T LET YOU

NOV. 2010

Don't Let Your Kids Be Normal

Gerry Fewster, Ph.D.

Centre for Child Honouring

Salt Spring Island

**All author profits for this book will be
donated to The Centre for Child Honouring.
More information can be found at
www.childhonouring.org**

For my daughter Cristine.

ACKNOWLEDGEMENTS

I would like to begin by acknowledging four remarkable teachers whose wisdom has inspired and sustained me over many years. Drs. Bennett Wong and Jock McKeen showed me how to open my heart and mind to embrace my own life in my own way. Dr. Jack Lee Rosenberg, the creator of Integrated Body Psychotherapy (IBP) offered me a framework in which that life could find its expression through my work and relationships, both professional and personal. The inimitable Virginia Satir, through her loving presence and consummate skills, taught me that I have absolutely nothing to hide.

For over fifty years I have shared a privileged professional pathway with many friends and colleagues who have provided me with the necessary stimulation and challenges to keep body, mind and spirit actively engaged. In particular I am profoundly grateful to those who have shared in the development of the ubiquitous profession known as Child and Youth Care. Dr. Sybille Artz, Dr. Jerry Beker, Michael Burns, Dr. Leon Fulcher, Brian Gannon, Dr. Thom Garfat, Dr. Kiaris Gharabaghi, Dr. Mark Krueger, Lorna McPherson, Dr. Henry Maier, Dr. Penny Parry, Jack Phelan, Kelly Shaw, Leanne Rose-Sladde, Dr. Carol Stuart, Dr. Karen VanderVen and Quinn Wilder are just few of the many pioneers who have committed themselves to enhancing the lives of young people around the world. Their work will never receive the recognition it deserves.

In writing this book, as with so many of my projects, I constantly turned to my long time buddy and mentor Dr. Mark Krueger for support and guidance. As always, it was given with characteristic clarity of mind and generosity of spirit.

In bringing the manuscript through its various developmental stages, I would like to thank Dr. Lynn Wytenbroek for her expert editorial work and Clarys Tirel for her thoughtful comments: and special appreciation to my dear niece, Jane Cummings, who helped to bring this work to the attention of 'thoughtful' parents. During the final writing phase, I was fortunate to receive the warm encouragement of Dr. David Chamberlain, a man whose work I have admired for so many years. His offer to write the Foreword rejuvenated me at a time when it was most needed. Then along came Julie Salisbury, a unique and dynamic force in the publishing business, who helped me to fine tune the manuscript and skillfully guided its passage through the inevitable contortions of birth. Publishing will never be the same.

When all is said and done, the only way to understand human relationships is through direct experience – *from the inside out*. With this clearly in mind, I want to express my deepest appreciation for every kid who taught me how to look beyond my pretensions of normality and seek out the mischievous rascal on the inside of us both. Through the course of this learning I have been aided and abetted by two of the most delightful deviants on the planet, Judith and our irrepressible daughter Cristine. I could not have asked for more.

Praise

"Gerry Fewster's latest book is a must read for anyone who is concerned about the world our children will inherit. In providing an in-depth practical guide for parents and professionals, Dr. Fewster challenges us to reconsider what human relationships are all about."

Jack Lee Rosenberg, Ph.D.
Founder and Director, Rosenberg-Kitaen International Institutes of Integrative Body Psychotherapy, Author of: *Body, Self & Soul* and *The Intimate Couple*.

"For many years, Gerry Fewster has been a leading figure in our field and his writings have had a dramatic impact on how many of us act, think and teach. In classic Fewster fashion, this new work shows us with examples, humor, creativity, and incredible depth of personal awareness and insight, how we might be in relationships with children, youth and families."

Mark Krueger, Ph.D.
Professor, University of Wisconsin, Director, Youth Work Learning Center, Milwaukee, Author of: *Nexus* and *Sketching Youth, Self and Youth Work*.

"Nobody exposes the plight and the potential of today's children more truthfully, eloquently and heart-fully."

Carol Matthews
Former Dean of Human Services and Community Education, Vancouver Island University, Author of: *The First Three Years of a Grandmother's Life*

Contents

FOREWORD

*D*on't Let Your Kids Be Normal is a rare, very personal work that caps a career of fifty years of personal and professional commitment to the well-being of children and their families. The author felt compelled to write this book because, throughout that time, he could find nothing in the existing literature that adequately reflected his personal experiences, thoughts and conclusions. In it he shares the deepest beliefs and convictions that were inspired by his own odyssey. He writes chapters that are conversations rather than lectures and offers options rather than prescriptions. Relationships are his business and, true to form, he invites his readers, whether parents or professionals, to join him on an urgent introspective journey that may yet assure the quality of *all* life on earth, our precious home planet.

University professor, master therapist, and notable director of an outstanding residential community for troubled youth, Gerry Fewster has been serving at the critical edge where dreams and realities collide and healing energies must be activated and perfected. He has been standing in that ever-so-common, yet sacred, space between adult and child. As you will soon discover, he invariably brings into this space his scholarly knowledge, dedicated curiosity, and a passionate faith in the creative inner Force that is the birthright of *human souls*.

Structurally, the seven "chapters" serve as staging grounds for approaching what he considers to be our greatest universal challenge – how to prepare our children to move with confidence and competence in a world filled with fear and uncertainty. Here the available evidence is carefully gathered and critically analyzed, until finally the author can articulate meaningful decisions, principles, and actions. The seven chapters are bound together by a brief Prologue in which he introduces himself and his intentions for the book; and an equally brief Epilogue for a final celebration of the surprising place our adult-child interactions occupy in shaping and re-shaping our lives on this planet.

When I first read this book I was pleasantly surprised to learn so much, so quickly about the author as a curious child, a struggling youth, compassionate therapist, and freethinking professor! These qualities were appealing and interesting to me; we were getting acquainted. Eventually, I realized I was getting all this information directly from Gerry because it was a key feature of how he writes, speaks, and interacts with people. Obviously, he was not trying to teach "self-disclosure" to me as a reader, but I saw that he not only "practices what he preaches" but he is constantly "modeling" a quality of dialogue known to improve relationships at any age! As you read ahead, I wonder if you will see what I saw.

Along the way you will encounter fascinating personal stories, original ideas, sharp and beautiful language, courageously independent thinking and knowledge broad and deep of the prenatal era of human development. Along with clear examples, practical exercises and poetry, you will become acquainted with a *host* of established experts he brings to every chapter.

If you are concerned about the future of our children, this book is bound to challenge many of your current assumptions and beliefs. If you are a thoughtful parent, or practicing professional, you will have the opportunity to explore new ways to create relationships that nurture the Self of both adult and child and uncover the untapped potential that lies beneath. The chances are that these approaches will be very different from what you learned in school or from your own parents, but I urge you to give them your serious consideration – time is of the essence.

David B. Chamberlain, Ph.D,
is a pioneer in birth psychology, and one of the founders of APPPAH
(Association for Pre- and Perinatal Psychology and Health),
Author of *The Mind of your Newborn Baby*

ABOUT GERRY FEWSTER

Gerry Fewster is an educator, writer and psychotherapist. For over twenty years he was Executive Director of one of Canada's largest privately operated treatment centers for troubled children and their families. He has held teaching positions at three universities and is currently Adjunct Associate Professor in the Department of Applied Psychology at the University of Calgary. Dr. Fewster has written extensively on children's mental health issues and is widely acknowledged for his 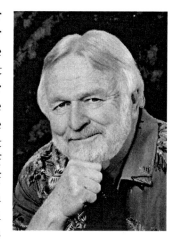 contributions to the development of Child and Youth Care across North America.

He was the editor of the *Journal of Child and Youth Care* for almost twenty years and editor of *Relational Child and Youth Care Practice*. Dr. Fewster has contributed over forty articles to professional journals and published a number of books including, *Being in child care: A journey into Self* (Haworth, N.Y., 1990) and *Ben and Jock: A biography* (Oolican, B.C., 2001).

He now lives on Vancouver Island where he and his partner Judith direct the Pacific North West Institute of Integrative Body Psychotherapy (IBP), one of ten international institutes dedicated to the advancement of human potential. Together the Fewster's maintain a private practice, specializing in relationship therapy.

PROLOGUE

L
ike so many projects in my life, this book turned out to be very different from its original conception. It began as a response to students in my Human Development classes who wanted to cover the terrain without having to scramble through the undergrowth in search of appropriate references and usable quotations. "Why don't you put it all together in one book?" they asked. "Because the content is changing all the time, depending on your curiosity and my ability to respond," I told them.

While my teaching methods were generally considered to be non-traditional, and the course outlines noted for their ambiguity, the fact is that the content prescribed in the university curriculum was faithfully covered. The only deviations were in the nature of the learning environment and in the stance taken toward the subject matter. In the first instance, my expectation was that students would become active participants in their own learning rather than passive recipients of packaged information. In particular, I encouraged them to revisit their own experiences of childhood for information and insights. In the second, I invited them to draw from this experience in a critical examination of the theories of developmental psychology, sharing not only their thoughts but also their feelings. My expressed agenda was for them to consider the possibility that human development is not a pre-determined trajectory of stages, norms and goals, but an infinite spectrum of possibilities in which we all have the inherent potential to create our own lives in our own way. In this highly personalized learning milieu, the only differences between me and my students was that I knew more about psychology, had many more years of experience in the field, and, of course, I was in charge of the class.

When I left my faculty position at the university, I was more interested in articulating this approach to learning than documenting the content of academic courses. The more I thought about it, the clearer it became that both aspects stem from the same basic beliefs, and each serves to reflect and reinforce the other. In my teaching, I had become convinced that education is not about filling empty minds but about stimulating those minds to think on their own behalf. Similarly, my years in professional practice had left me in no doubt that lives cannot be fixed from the outside; they can only be re-created from the inside. The underlying belief is that we are all at the center of our own lives, and we learn whatever we happen to be searching for. The attempt to bring the subject matter and the learner - the knowledge and the knower - together within an integrated conceptual framework seemed like an exciting challenge.

But, much as I loved the teaching, once I set about to the task of writing, I found it difficult to sustain my enthusiasm. The root of the problem was that my most basic beliefs about human potential seemed to be completely at odds with the current reality. Only a fool would speculate about moving to higher levels of consciousness when our flagrant disregard for our planet is dragging us back to the most basic developmental imperative – physical survival. How could anybody reasonably argue that empathy and compassion are innate characteristics in every human infant when over a third of the world's population is being decimated by disease and starvation? And who in his or her right mind would talk about our inherent relatedness when the distribution of wealth and resources has become so polarized that the values and structures that once held together our families, communities and nations have been stretched beyond recognition?

All this was bad enough, but when I considered the reasons for our disarray, I found myself totally out of step with the popular versions of consensual reality. I have never seriously considered the human condition as being imposed on us by ruthless dictators, religious fanatics, power-hungry politicians, or corporate criminals. However ugly these spectres might appear, they are merely foils, convenient projections of our collective fears and individual irresponsibility. We may set out to destroy them through military or ideological cleansing, but until we recognize them as our own creations, we will simply replace them and continue to recycle our psychic waste.

Our overriding challenge isn't ideological, political, or even environmental – it is essentially developmental. We can talk all we want about creating a more caring and harmonious world, but this will never happen until we learn how to be with one another as curious, caring, and compassionate beings. This isn't about inventing a new world order; it's about personal awareness and transformation, beginning with our most primary relationships. On the one hand, we can sit back and wait for divine intervention or for evolutionary influences to move us to the next developmental stage. On the other, we can choose to see ourselves as participants in that process, recognize our potentials and take responsibility for our own destiny. Given the urgency of our predicament, I consider this to be a much more life-affirming strategy.

The more I pushed myself to write about these things, the more I became aware of my own complicity. Apart from brief episodes of adolescent defiance, I have never been an active agent for social change, and have remained cynical about how easily the most innocent of human values and expressions can become corrupted into impersonal political and religious ideologies. But the justifications I have always used to live within the protected relationships of my own life, while allowing the universe to 'unfold as it should,' were beginning to wear thin. A growing sense of negligence and irresponsibility, fueled by unsettling questions about my own integrity, urged me to think again about my tenuous place in this troubled world. If I am part of the unfolding order, then I can do no less than acknowledge my part in its creation, not in the service of my conscience but as an affirmation of my consciousness. If I have the option to act upon that awareness, then perhaps I should do so, not as an agent of change but simply as a way of being.

I mean it when I say that writing this book has changed my life. With only myself as witness, I was free to suspend the demands of my ego and listen to my own voice. Even my most sacrosanct beliefs could be unwrapped and re-examined without fear of recrimination. Nevertheless, my unsettled and insecure mind would frequently take up its familiar stance, wondering how I would be judged by anyone who might read my words. Time and again, I reminded myself to remain grounded in my own experience, urging my mind to accept my feelings and emotions as legitimate contributors to the exercise. In many ways, the experience was quite similar to my university classes, with me as the solitary learner.

Whenever I examine my experience in this way, it becomes abundantly clear that the central issues in my life have always revolved around relationships, my search for connection. Since I have chosen to spend so much of my life around children and young people, it seems reasonable to assume I have something to learn with and from them. In so many ways, this book is the product of that learning through over fifty years of personal exploration and professional practice. If this turns out to be useful to anyone else, I will be delighted.

As a final note, I would like to make a general statement about the format of this book. As a general rule, books dealing with psychological matters fall into one of two distinctive categories. On the one hand, there is the traditional theoretical and empirical textbook, designed for academics, students and practicing professionals. On the other, we have that plethora of literature, known as 'Pop Psychology,' written for less 'serious,' and presumably less 'sophisticated,' readers who are more concerned about what's happening in their own lives. My intention in blending these two forms is to assist general readers to understand what the 'experts' have to say, and to urge the 'experts' to test out their theories in the human laboratory of everyday life. I believe the time has come for us all to think deeply about what it means to be fully human, with ourselves, each other and, most urgently, with our children.

Gerry Fewster, 2008

CHAPTER ONE

Leaving Home

Since you've picked up this book and managed to get this far into the text, it's likely you have some interest in those mysterious formative years between conception and adulthood when so much is supposed to happen and so many things seem to go wrong. If you're like most adults drawn to this topic, you will be looking for something you don't already know - a startling new theory, a new perspective on parenting, or maybe the latest prescriptions for getting kids to behave as they should. Hopefully, there's enough good stuff in this book to hold your interest, but my intention in writing is somewhat more ambitious.

My primary purpose is to invite you to take another look at childhood and adolescence from a unique perspective – your own. In this cause, I will draw upon the ideas and experiences of others, but my desire is that you will use your own experience as the critical perspective. This isn't only about sifting through old childhood memories or seeking

Preoccupied with our day-by-day obligations, aspirations and fears, we have come to think of childhood as a bother-some develop-mental phase and consider children as adults-in-training.

some version of the 'child within'. My invitation is for you to bring all your adult curiosity, experiences and faculties to the task. In the final analysis, you may decide to modify your assumptions or generate even more support for your existing beliefs.

Having spent much of my life working with 'problem' kids, I'm convinced that most parents, professionals and academics are no longer interested in, or even curious about, that time when we all struggled to come to terms with the world created and inhabited by our adult caretakers. Preoccupied with our day-by-day obligations, aspirations and fears, we have come to think of childhood as a bothersome developmental phase and consider children as adults-in-training. Our overriding concern is that they should learn the ropes as quickly as possible in order to match our expectations, whatever they happen to be. If we really want them to stay ahead of the game, we read books on child development, attend parenting classes, send them to the best schools, and reward them for fulfilling our ambitions. In other words, we drag them away from the natural agendas and authentic experiences of childhood, and if they submit without too much of a hassle, we reward them with the latest gadgets and trips to Disneyland. If they stumble, we urge them to press on. If they stay down, we up the ante with additional loaded rewards, punishments and deprivations. If they rebel, we resort to our tired methods of discipline, and if nothing seems to do the trick, we call in the experts. For all this, we demand their attention, their compliance, their respect and their love.

Of course, you may consider this to be a biased, or even cynical view conjured up by an aging and jaded people-worker who has spent far too long hanging around crazy kids and fractured families. That is certainly your right, but I want to assure you that I am not trying to point the finger of blame in any particular direction. I realize most parents and teachers are well intended and sincerely believe they act in the best interests of the children in their care. I also happen to believe, that at the very core, we are all caring and compassionate human beings. My humble intention is to offer some possible alternatives to our ways of being with children and young people. In my experience, the old ways are no longer viable.

I believe the time has come for us to seriously reconsider the notion that the central task of parenting is to teach children how to live and succeed in a world we once knew or thought we knew. Even among the most privileged nations and groups, this world is no longer a place that offers any sense of safety and security for the next generation. For better or for worse, we have created a reality that detaches us from ourselves, from each other, and from a planet that struggles to sustain our indulgences. We

> *In this state of confusion, it is deceptive and ultimately futile to impose what we learned from our parents onto our children.*

have set out to systematically dismantle the traditional structures of family, community, nation and culture and, in this new liberalism, the time-tested parenting values of discipline, obedience and respect for elders have become an ineffective anachronism.

While these old values and beliefs may have been less than ideal, and in some cases were downright repressive, they at least constrained our discordant ambitions and served to define our place in the scheme of things. More specifically, they told us how we should relate to one another – leader to follower, employer to employee, husband to wife, teacher to student, parent to child. But, since we have chosen to 'liberate' ourselves from the power-based traditions and institutions that held these roles together, we now face the challenge of redefining who we really are, and where we stand in relation to one another. In this state of confusion, it is deceptive and ultimately futile to impose what we learned from our parents onto our children.

So what prevents us from moving forward to create a world that offers meaning, purpose and fulfillment for ourselves, and a desirable future for our children? The simple answer is fear. There is no place on this planet where anyone can feel secure about the present or the future and, let's face it, short of divine intervention or visitors from space, there's nobody 'out there' who will come along to look after us. When children sense our insecurity, we can always point to external causes; from the terrorism of Al Qaeda to the melting of the polar ice caps. Through our multitude of unresolved fears, we pass on the message that the world is a precarious and potentially hostile place.

The only way we will ever overcome the helplessness that keeps us fearful and frozen is to look inward and discover that we, the creators, have what it takes to re-create the world as we would want it to be.

However real these threats may be, I believe the source of our dis-ease lies more on the inside than the outside. We can continue to attack and destroy the external enemies, but until we come to realize that these are of our own creation, we will continue to invent new monsters in the forlorn hope that their destruction will bring about the security and freedom we long for. What we fail to see is that our battle is essentially against ourselves. The only way we will ever overcome the helplessness that keeps us fearful and frozen is to look inward and discover that we, the creators, have what it takes to re-create the world as we would want it to be. The alternatives are to lash out in frustration and anger, transcend into the cosmic ether, or sink into apathy and denial. The critical question is not what we tell our children about the world, but what we are able and willing to tell them about ourselves. This is the information they will need to do things differently. It's no longer about educating them - it's a matter of survival.

Grow up or Give up?

At some point in our lives, most of us went through that unsettling stage when we demanded our independence on the outside while, on the inside, we were riddled with doubt and confusion. On the one hand, we wanted freedom; on the other, we knew we were still dependent upon the support of our caretakers. To make the break, some of us turned our adult providers into the enemy, agents of repression, and openly rebelled. Some of us turned our anxieties inward, complying on the surface while swallowing our anger and resentment. Feeling unsure, powerless and alone, most of us sought solace in the company of other lost souls and created our own transitory sense of security. In order to move on, we must eventually come to realize that what we are looking for is not on the outside at all. To take charge of our lives and to become self-responsible, we must discover our uniqueness and our relatedness, and come to know that we can make our own decisions without losing either along the way. We refer to this critical phase of our individual development as 'adolescence'.

To become self-responsible, we must discover our uniqueness and our relatedness, and come to know that we can make our own decisions without losing either along the way.

As individuals, many of us might claim we have made the transition into the conscious and self-responsible state of adulthood. This may be so, but it seems clear to me that, as a species, we are still struggling with our collective adolescence. Rather than face the prospect of moving on, we have created a compelling deluge of external political, economic, social and ideological reasons to remain stuck in our confused and dependent state. Meanwhile, technology is expanding our global awareness and the consequences of our developmental stagnation are giving rise to a growing sense of disillusionment and discontent. Old beliefs are falling by the wayside, to be replaced by cynicism and helplessness. Developmentally we are urged to move on, but the freedom we seek cannot be gained without that critical shift from relying upon the old sources of security to embracing the uncertainty of whatever lies beyond.

This is unexplored territory, and while there are certainly those who have taken the first tentative steps into the unknown, their voices are seldom heard above the rabble. These are not the charismatic leaders and experts we have come to demand and depend upon. They have no packaged solutions for our discontent, no vision of what might be, and no assurances we will find what we're looking for. These are the risk-takers who know only their own humility and seek to understand whatever stands before them. They are leaders without followers. Our challenge is not to walk behind them, but to join them by drawing upon the resources and potentials that lie within every one of us; the ability to see, to hear, to make choices and to relate to ourselves and others as caring, compassionate and responsible human beings. These are not conditions that can be learned and imposed from the outside or expressed in the name of some social, political or religious ideology: they are the basic ingredients of our humanness that can only be discovered on the inside and expressed through our relationships with one another.

My simple proposition is that children who are fortunate enough to be raised under such influences will feel welcomed, nurtured and secure in the world. Acknowledged and respected for who they are, they will seek the same qualities within themselves and others. Such children will have the resources to move confidently through the turmoil and confusion that is their dubious legacy. Regardless of whatever might be taking place around them, they will always have access to a place of security on the inside – their own indomitable sense of Self. Drawing from their own inner resources, rather than external prescriptions, they will be able to create relationships that reflect the essence of their humanity. In other words, they will leave the transitory shelters of their parents to discover a home within themselves. With our support and encouragement, such children will have what it takes to change the world.

> *We cannot give our children what we ourselves don't have ... Our challenge is to learn how to re-parent ourselves.*

So what prevents us from raising our children this way? Well, as I will say many times and in many ways throughout this book, we cannot give our children what we ourselves don't have. As adults, we can no longer look to our parents to take us to this inside place; the onus is upon us to find our own way home, to discover, nurture, and create our own sense of Self. Our challenge is to learn how to re-parent ourselves, to give to ourselves what we didn't get when we were growing up.

But first, we must let our own parents off the hook. They are not responsible for the choices we make as adults. For the most part they passed on whatever they learned from their caretakers, for better or for worse. To acknowledge their efforts and move on is the first step we must take toward our own individuation and self-responsibility. Then, as we begin to discover the resources within ourselves, every revelation and every insight offers a potential gift, to ourselves and to those around us. Our fears don't disappear, but they are mediated by an inner knowing that, whatever the circumstances, we belong in this place, an integral part of the whole. Above all, this makes it possible to share with our children what they most need; the undisguised truth of what it means to be an adult and a conscious human being struggling to live in a fractured and fearful world.

But can we really expect young children to understand the complexity of adult life? I think so. In the first place, our lives are not that complex. Once stripped of the mind's pretensions, our hopes and fears turn out to be remarkably simple – not unlike waiting for Santa Claus, making friends, and fretting about the monsters in the bedroom closet. Learning how to access and communicate our inner experiences in a way kids can understand is our challenge, not theirs. Nature has ensured that, even before birth, children are able to let us know about their inner experiences. We don't need words or concepts to understand what they have to say. We understand because, beneath the layers of thoughts and language that complicate our lives, the same wordless system of communication is still alive and active in all of us. We may refer to this as intuition or energetic connection, and whether we are aware of it or not, this system continues to express our inner experience to whoever happens to be tuned in to the frequency. And on this waveband, children are very adept, attentive and non-censoring receivers.

Understanding ourselves and relating to others are complementary aspects of the same developmental process. By taking the risk to know and share our authentic experiences, we become secure enough on the inside to hear the truth of others, even when such revelations are not to our liking. For example, much as we might want our children to love us unconditionally, a child's sense of loving is firmly conditional and can quickly turn to anger, or even hate, when his or her immediate wants are not being satisfied. If these intense feelings are unacceptable to the parent, the child represses them. Yet, as Alice Miller articulates so clearly in her book *Prisoners of Childhood*, such 'ugly' feelings are essential to the child's development of Self. If repressed, they are subsequently manifested in the form of emotional insecurity, depression and the creation of a 'false self" to replace the authentic Self.

Parents who maintain a solid sense of Self, can hear and acknowledge these feelings without censorship while remaining open and curious about their child's experiences. Additionally, children who are not afraid to reveal their own inner world, remain open and curious about themselves and others. With the parent leading the way, the learning that takes place between adult and child is

I am not suggesting, however, that we should abandon our parental and adult responsibilities to teach children about how to live in this world.

respectful, mutual and profoundly bonding. In my own practice, I have never worked with a child who, having shared some aspect of personal 'truth,' has not taught me something of value about himself or herself, about childhood and, in the most astonishing ways, about me.

There is no question that what I am proposing fundamentally redefines the traditional parent-child, and even the adult-child, relationship. I am not suggesting, however, that we should abandon our parental and adult responsibilities to teach children about how to live in this world. They need to understand what the expectations are and what values, if any, lie behind our beliefs and our

*Nothing is ever
lost through the
simple authenticity
of being human.*

actions. They need the security of knowing that there is somebody out there who will say "no" when their wants are turned into demands. This is essential preparation for the time when they are ready to take responsibility for creating their own expectations, and adapting their own values.

The difference here is that the external authority becomes known to the child as an accessible human being, complete with all the doubts, fears, hopes and dreams that live within us all. Nothing is ever lost through the simple authenticity of being human. The days when parents and adults could consider children as empty vessels to be molded into some version of what a 'good' child should look like are over. Unfortunately, the rules that governed this form of parenting are often replaced by arbitrary expectations that children should demonstrate their love and respect for their parents through their behavior, academic performance and compliant attitude. When this fails, as it so often does, the problem is seen to lie within the child. Of course it isn't the child that needs the attention, but it will remain this way until those of us who live and work with children realize that it is we who must attend to the next phase of our own development. Essentially, the time has come for us to grow up.

The Foundations of Fear

So, what are we really afraid of? If the next stage in our evolution directs our attention inward, all we will discover is our Selves, our own authenticity. Yet, for most of us, such logic offers only flimsy assurance, and those who contemplate the prospect often report being 'scared' of what they might find on the inside: others decide from the outset that they simply 'don't want to know.'

It's easy to dismiss such fears as irrational, but experience suggests they are not. The revelations and insights of self-discovery are their own reward, but such knowledge comes at a price. Each step along the way we find ourselves confronting the myths and monuments we have created in our attempts to assure ourselves of our permanent place in the scheme of things. Under such scrutiny, many of our most sacrosanct 'truths' dissolve into illusions; totally incapable of supporting the hypotheses we have always taken for granted. Financial wealth, material possessions, social status, personal power, certificates of achievement, and the regalia of office, turn out to be little more than masks to conceal the emptiness on the inside. On the outside, our social institutions, structures and ideologies begin to appear as feeble fortresses in our constant battle with the eternal order. But the most disturbing part of all comes when we begin to realize that even the beliefs we hold about ourselves, our individuality, identity and personality, are also illusions – defenses constructed to protect us from the truth of who we really are and where we really fit into nature's design.

> *The most disturbing part of all comes when we begin to realize that even the beliefs we hold about ourselves, our individuality, identity and personality, are also illusions – defenses constructed to protect us from the truth of who we really are and where we really fit into nature's design.*

In this sense, we are like kids who know when it's time to leave home, yet balk at the prospect. We challenge the prevailing 'truths' but have neither the experience nor the wisdom to replace them. The questions we ask are essentially the same: if I am not who I thought I was, then who am I? Who will look after me if Mom, Dad, the

President, and the Good Fairy are no longer viable options? Why would I set out on a journey when the route is uncharted and the destination is unknown?

Rather than respond to such questions with curiosity and courage, our collective inclination has been to opt for one of the two familiar 'adolescent adjustment reactions.' The first is to rebel – to transform our fear into anger and hold the rest of world responsible for our discontent. The second is to retreat – to turn our anxiety against ourselves and sink into various forms of confusion and depression. It is no coincidence that aggression and depression have become rampant in all societies where the values of individualism and materialism have come to define the social context. A third, and by far the most dangerous reaction, is to regress into infant dependency and lay ourselves at the feet of some all-powerful authority – terrestrial or otherwise – in the forlorn hope that someone may take pity on us and save us from ourselves.

As children, it was virtually impossible for us to remain curious and fearful at the same time but, as adults, we have the ability to do just that.

From a developmental point of view, the only viable option is to come to terms with our individual mortal impermanence and reclaim that unique human quality that we all brought into this world – curiosity. As children, it was virtually impossible for us to remain curious and fearful at the same time but, as adults, we have the ability to do just that. We also have the capacity to be rational and responsible in dealing with whatever we happen to discover. Simply because we find something is not to our liking doesn't mean we must destroy it before moving on. However dilapidated the house, and however dysfunctional the family, we all need the security of a home-base when the going gets tough. Our primary task is not to demolish what is, but to recognize things for what they are and understand why we created them in the first place. Then, as we come to realize we have options, in both our personal lives and our collective creations, we can begin to make those changes that support our individual and collective well being. We cannot immediately change the world for the benefit of our children, but through our curiosity and our courage, we can begin to lay the foundation for a more caring, compassionate and life-affirming future.

This is a future that can never be planned or predicted. The twin virtues of curiosity and courage will undoubtedly take us to places that lie beyond the scope of our imagination. Amid all the uncertainty, only one thing is for sure. At some point, we will find ourselves drawn to a place of anguish that lies deep within every human life. This is often considered to be a confrontation with death, the certainty of our own mortality. However, I believe it's more than that. The inevitability of physical death is a known reality, but the termination of our inner life, when the Self as we know it ceases to be, is a prospect few are inclined to consider. Consider it we must. This is a place where we stand naked and alone, bereft of all assurances and staring into the blackness of our own extinction – a 'somebody' about to become a 'nobody'. Here there are no gurus or saviours reaching across the void promising preservation' or salvation.

The English novelist John Fowles has called this place of non-existence the "Nemo" and the terror it invokes is often referred to as "the dark night of the soul." Whatever beliefs have served to assuage our fears, and however much we have filled the void with earthly deeds and acquisitions, there is no escape. To step purposefully into this place requires supreme courage; to remain open to whatever we find there and move on is the ultimate act of faith. This is not the faith to blindly follow what others have told us, but the confidence that comes from acknowledging our own existence. What might we find beyond the darkness? My own belief is that beneath the fear we will find our authentic being, although that will always remain a matter of faith.

If this seems like a less than heavenly conclusion to our developmental journey on this planet, there are two factors that might make the prospect more tolerable. First is the recognition that this is not our first confrontation with the incomprehensible darkness. 'Object Relations' theorists tell us that our earliest experiences of life are a constant struggle for survival no matter how much our parents strive to make us feel safe and secure. Any separation from mother (or the 'mother object'), however fleeting, evokes the universal terror of abandonment, and a primal knowing that, without her presence we will surely die. More recently, researchers in the field of Pre- and Perinatal Psychology have proposed that, at a deep somatic level, we experience this anguish even before birth, whenever our life-affirming synchronicity with mother is momentarily suspended. Yet such separation is essential and must be successfully managed for the natural process of development to occur.

My own belief is that beneath the fear we will find our authentic being, although that will always remain a matter of faith.

In the world of Object Relations, the ever-increasing distance between mother and child is known as 'transitional space'. In early childhood, we fill this void with a variety of objects, including other people, to ward off the terror until mother returns. The term 'transitional object' refers to those 'mother substitutes' that give us a sense of contact and control when we feel abandoned and helpless. As we become more independent, and our survival seems more assured, the fear of being abandoned slips beneath the surface. But it never goes away. Even in adulthood that same anguish surges back whenever our 'reality' is challenged and our sense of Self begins to fall apart. To protect ourselves from this life-threatening

It is the certainty of uncertainty that challenges our minds to reach out, to create new meanings and conditions for life on this planet.

experience, many of us continue to create transitional objects. In some cases we even endow them with human characteristics. I am embarrassed to acknowledge that my old long-case clock "Tom" and my little red car "Millie" are personal examples.

The second fragile assurance is the knowledge that the Nemo is both the source and the product of our own imagination – a distinctively human creation that stems from our ability to contemplate the termination of our lives and speculate about what might, or might not, lie beyond. It is the certainty of uncertainty that challenges our minds to reach out, to create new meanings and conditions for life on this planet. It is real in the same way our lives are real, and if we are to move toward higher levels of consciousness and freedom, it must be faced and understood for what it is. This will not take away the fear, but this is not the object of the exercise. Our task is to recognize its rightful place in creating the tensions that are essential to the evolution of human life. Then, and only then, will we cease to project our deepest fears onto each other and onto a planet that isn't equipped to take it any longer. The alternative is to continue to look outside and place ourselves in the hands of the gurus and power brokers; whether they are dictators, fundamentalists, corporate executives or democratically elected officials promising us freedom and a better future for all. As Churchill could well have said, "Some freedom, some future!"

The Fearful and the Fixers

Meanwhile, what can we say to our children about this state of affairs? How can we explain a world in turmoil and a planet on the brink of social and ecological breakdown? If this is the brave new world we have created for them to inherit, then we need look no further to explain why so many of our kids are numbing out, dropping out, shooting up, or simply telling us to go to Hell. In her book *The Continuum Concept*, published in 1975, Jean Liedloff tells us how children come into this world with an innate sense of what they need and what is 'right' for their own development and well-being. By the same thesis, we might conclude they also know when things are terribly 'wrong' and, no matter how much we try to assure them otherwise with empty gestures of a false security, our duplicity is reflected in our confusion and in every move we make.

We have chosen to tag them with meaningless labels conjured up by the guardians of the old morality who prescribe what is, and what is not, 'normal'.

In their unsophisticated way, our children, from infancy through adolescence, are showing us what we have chosen not to see, and true to form, we resent them for their naive honesty. This is not the place for statistics, but it's abundantly clear that, across the supposedly 'advanced' nations, the number of kids identified as being problems to themselves and others is simply staggering. Rather than look into this unsettling mirror, we have chosen to tag them with meaningless labels conjured up by the guardians of the old morality who prescribe what is, and what is not, 'normal'. Just as we look to our leaders to define the new order, so we look to the experts to tell us what's wrong and how we should deal with the problem.

The solutions are not working and children are 'speaking back' in ever-increasing numbers, using whatever means are available. Unless some fundamental change occurs, there will be even more confused, depressed and angry youth out there for us to worry about. Parents and teachers will continue to demand more from the experts and pharmaceutical companies, while the detached adults - those who receive their information from the popular media – will become even more convinced that kids are a threat

Yet despite the evidence, we continue to believe the problem lies within individual youngsters and after labeling them accordingly, we set out to treat their pathology.

to their personal security and society at large. In the labeling game, this is a condition known as 'pedophobia', defined as a generalized fear of young people.

What can we say about a society that has become fearful of its own children? Or, more introspectively, what is the nature of the fear we project onto those who look to us for security, support and guidance? The one thing we can be assured of is that this is a self-fulfilling belief. Tagged as objects of failure, deviance, and potential terrorism, kids with no other sense of identity will inhabit these roles and claim their power by playing upon our fears. In other words, they become the monsters in our secret closet. Alternatively, and more tragically, others will internalize such attributions and turn against themselves. Do we need to look any further to account for the dramatic escalation of self-inflicted harm among children and adolescents? Across affluent nations, drug and alcohol abuse, physical violations like 'cutting' and 'slashing,' eating disorders such as anorexia nervosa and, of course, attempted suicide, have become commonplace wherever young people are to be found. Only twenty years ago, when I ran a large treatment center for severely emotionally disturbed children, such self-destructive behaviors were relatively rare, now they are routinely accepted as the presenting symptoms. Yet despite the evidence, we continue to believe the problem lies within individual youngsters and after labeling them accordingly, we set out to treat their pathology.

Children in need of help became 'cases' that needed treatment and the pharmaceutical industry reveled in the new market it had worked so diligently to create.

As a professional, I have made my own contribution to this dehumanizing mythology. Time and again I've offered false assurances to parents who wanted to hear they were not to 'blame' for their kid's problems. Making no distinction between blame and responsibility, they accepted my counsel without question and, in most cases, were more than willing to look to me for the solutions. I was never completely at ease with this arrangement, but in the service of my ego and my income, I counseled myself to go along with the charade. The seriousness of my hypocrisy did not hit home until the early 1980's when tagging kids with meaningless psychiatric and psychological labels became the order of the day.

The Labeling Game

Over the next decade, the number of new syndromes and disorders escalated dramatically, and it became rare for me to work with any youngster who wasn't suffering from some malady described and classified in the psychiatric diagnostic manuals. Children in need of help became 'cases' that needed treatment and the pharmaceutical industry reveled in the new market it had worked so diligently to create. By the turn of the century the system had accommodated to this mythology to the point where it was almost impossible for any young person to receive professional help without some standardized label assigned by a duly authorized representative of the industry. Parents and teachers were happy to be off the hook, professionals basked in their status as experts, and the profits of the drug companies soared to unprecedented heights.

To an alarming degree, even the kids have bought into the mythology. For many, it's so much more acceptable to be suffering from 'Oppositional Defiance Disorder' than to accept personal responsibility for telling a teacher to "fuck off". It's also no surprise that many kids are more than happy to take pills to numb out the confusion and anguish they feel on the inside. Predictably, they have also been quick to realize that prescription drugs are profitable commodities that can be marketed to eager consumers in schools, youth clubs and on street corners everywhere.

How much more of our power must we give away before we completely hand our bodies over to the physicians, our minds to the psychiatrists, our values to the moralists, and our Souls to whatever god seems to offer the best hope for salvation?

In other words, we seem to have a neatly woven system that appears to meet the requirements of all who participate. For most of us, the absolution of responsibility for both our problems and their solutions is symptomatic of the modern way, whether we are talking about kids, computers, our health, or U.S. foreign policy. Yet, however convenient this stance may seem, it lies at the very core of the feelings of alienation and helplessness that fuel our growing discontent. How much more of our power must we give away before we completely hand our bodies over to the physicians, our minds to the psychiatrists, our values to the moralists, and our Souls to whatever god seems to offer the best hope for salvation?

Unless we find the courage to identify the sources of our lingering discontent, we will continue to project it onto our children. The more we relinquish authority over our own lives, the more we seek to demonstrate our power over the lives of others, and since children are dependent upon us for their survival, they have always been prime targets for our stifled ambitions. Claiming them as 'our own flesh and blood,' we look upon them as extensions of ourselves, living assurance of our immortality. What we want from them is not the expression of their unique qualities and potentials as human beings, but their unquestioning obedience to our cause. The less we believe in ourselves, the more we demand their unconditional respect and conformity as a shallow substitute for our missing sense of being. If they fail to fulfill these expectations, as they always will, we have only the power of external authority to bring them into line. Sometimes we call this 'discipline' and sometimes we call it 'treatment' or 'therapy'.

Fixing the problem as quickly and inexpensively as possible from the outside is the service most parents seem to want and what most professionals attempt to deliver.

Let's Play Doctor

One of the many problems of handing our kids over to the experts is that very few professionals are actually prepared, or even trained, to create the kind of relationships that attend to the inner life of their young clientele. Even if such individuals can be found, developing a relationship based upon curiosity, mutual understanding and respect takes far too long, and costs considerably more than most of us are prepared to pay.

Fixing the problem as quickly and inexpensively as possible from the outside is the service most parents seem to want and what most professionals attempt to deliver.

The broader issue that discourages professionals from creating meaningful relationships with their clients is that most of us have been trained to think of ourselves as 'scientists' striving to remain 'objective' in diagnosing problems, creating solutions and measuring observable outcomes. Enamored by the achievements of modern medicine, we have been encouraged to consider our clients as objects to be studied according to a set of pre-existing rules and procedures. Based upon this understanding, we are taught how to intervene in the person's social, mental, emotional and spiritual life in order to treat the identified problem, in much the same way as a physician might treat a case of measles. We readily adopt medical concepts and terminology, describing our work as 'clinical' and using various forms of 'intervention,' 'treatment' and 'therapy' to attain our objectives. Failure to bring about the desired outcome might be attributed to three factors: insufficient data, misapplied or inadequate theory; and faulty application. In its purest and most sophisticated form, this model has become known as 'psychotherapy'.

When it comes to creating personal relationships, this so-called 'medical model' is an abomination. To be 'objective,' professionals are supposed to bracket-off their own personal thoughts and feelings and focus upon treating the identified problem or 'condition'. The purpose of the exercise is not to *be with* the other person but to *do something to* him or her. By the same token, the inner life of the patient, or client, is generally discounted, unless such personal experiences can be conveniently classified and slotted into the preferred theory of the practitioner. Once identified as a 'case' of something or other, the person is removed from the equation and the treatment can begin. The recipient can now be assured that the problem is not of his or her own making and that the professional has the power to make it all better. Both participate in the same absurd illusion. Both are equally irresponsible and deluded – the client for believing that he or she is a victim and the professional for believing that he or she has the power to fix someone else's life. They are co-conspirators; each using the other against the fear of the Nemo. If either were to come clean, to dismantle the illusion, the contract would fall apart at the seams.

While the medical model fits well within the technological age, the current state of our planet serves as a grim reminder that our current scientific principles and practices have serious limitations. When it comes to understanding ourselves, they have been an abysmal failure. In the field of psychology, we have attempted to detach ourselves from ourselves in order to understand ourselves – a ridiculous proposition when you really think about it. We have turned ourselves into objects, and from this shallow perspective, we created a distorted mirror, a reflection that strips us of our unique experiences, our individuality, our volition and our humanity. Fortunately proponents of Quantum Theory are now offering us a radically different view of the universe, our planet and our place in the scheme of things. Through their window we get our first tantalizing glimpses of human beings as conscious, purposeful and essentially unpredictable elements within the cosmos – active participants in nature's process. This is a story that is only just beginning to unfold in the face of powerful resistance from those who have been trained to believe otherwise. Meanwhile, the science we have come to know and trust continues to portray us as biologically determined organisms responding to whatever our bodies demand and our brain dictates. This is why we need the experts to tell us about who we are and to manipulate the odds on our behalf, even though most of us have no idea what the hell they're talking about.

If you're familiar with the most recent psychiatric diagnostic manuals, you will know there's no end to this insidious nonsense. Since all aspects of life are connected in some way, any grouping of factors can be turned into a disorder without a disease, a syndrome without a cause, or a brain without a mind. By scientific standards however, the only explanations that really measure up are those that would have us enslaved by our own biological and neurological processes - the 'new frontier' they call it. Through the microscope, or its modern day equivalents, our roots are supposedly revealed, our experiences explained and our destinies predicted. Whether or not you choose to accept or challenge the conclusions of the experts, there can be no question that our behavior, our thoughts and our emotions can be fundamentally changed through the chemical manipulation of our bodies and brains. The scientific evidence is compelling and seductive. It's compelling because those who understand it are invested in the old clockwork models of science, and it's seductive because it offers those who don't a solid 'scientific' reason to avoid the daunting prospect of having to seek the 'truth' within the laboratory of their own lives.

This isn't about contradicting a Nobel Prize winning neuro-physicist in his or her own specialized domain. Only a small handful of people would be able and prepared to pose such a challenge. The only question we can put to such an eminent scholar is, "If you believe this is what my life is all about, do you also believe this about your life?" Whatever the answer, the questions to be asked are not 'scientific' in the traditional sense, and the answers are not to be found in the data generated in some esoteric field of study, scientific or otherwise. These are questions we must ask of ourselves and, as the experts within our own lives, we must also be ready to make sense of our

*From the moment
of our conception
to the moment of our
departure, our most
enduring and pervasive
developmental need
is for connection
with others.*

findings, constantly refining our enquiry in a disciplined and systematic manner. In this, we all have access to the same incredible instrument of enquiry and analysis that evolution has bestowed upon us – the neo-cortex. If we are to break loose from the psychological and religious shackles that keep us apart from each other, and ourselves we can no longer afford to allow this gift of evolution to remain idle in its packing case. It will not operate unless we instruct it to do so, and it will not provide us with the information we need until we have the commitment to ask the questions and the courage to consider the answers.

The Relationship Crucible

The central paradox in the development of the Self is that we cannot individuate alone. We are human only to the degree that we recognize the same human qualities in others. Without you, there can be no "me" to be known, and without each other, we have no reason to be in this world. From the moment of our conception to the moment of our departure, our most enduring and pervasive developmental need is for connection with others. As we move from the dependency of childhood, and our emerging Self becomes increasingly central in our lives, our relational aspirations gradually shift from the satisfaction of basic survival needs to that of creating a place for ourselves in the world as conscious, self-directed and relational human beings. This is a life-long process through which our authentic Self seeks to move toward increasingly higher levels of definition, integration and expression. It is an adventure beset with many obstacles but, I venture to suggest, this is exactly as it should be. In overcoming the frustration of the interruptions and the pain of the injuries, the Self gains its inner strength and the necessary volition to become an active agent in an otherwise obdurate world.

Relationships are both the context and the vehicle for this process, and our constant challenge is to find ways to be involved with others without losing our Selves along the way. Moving beyond Mommy and Daddy, we all seek at least one special relationship in which we can be seen and heard for who we really are as separate and unique beings. This isn't the pursuit of some hazy romantic dream; it's created purposefully over time through moment-by-moment exchanges in which each participant takes the risk to reveal Self to the Other. When this occurs between those we call 'parents,' the children are the unconditional beneficiaries. When such relationships are brought into connection with others, they establish the foundation for the creation of families and communities held together through the recognition of our undeniable and universal relatedness. This is the pathway of individuation, the convoluted trail that takes us from the dependency of childhood through the growing pains of adolescence and urges us on toward self-directed re-connection.

For most of us, this is no stroll in the park. However much we believe we have successfully separated from our parents or childhood caregivers, our individuation is not accomplished by the simple act of leaving home. There is still much to be done, and whatever we have learned, or not learned, is taken into our subsequent relationships. As adults, we can always adjust our behaviors in response to the other person, but unless we are aware of the missing pieces, chances are, we will look to our current relationships to give us what we didn't get in our early years. The trouble is that these people are not our parents, and no matter how much they might try, they can never satisfy our residual childhood longings. Unless we recognize that these are things we must now give to ourselves, the authenticity and intimacy we are looking for in our relationships will remain smothered beneath a perpetual overlay of demands, deception and resentment. In short, we are well and truly stuck.

In order to separate from our parents and move to higher levels of individuation, we must become aware of the interruptions and injuries in our early developmental history, and take full ownership for whatever remedial work needs to be done.

In order to separate from our parents and move to higher levels of individuation, we must become aware of the interruptions and injuries in our early developmental history, and take full ownership for whatever remedial work needs to be done. This alone is more than sufficient reason for us to turn our curiosity inward and re-examine the experiences of our childhood. To some extent we can do this by retrieving the memories of those early years. The problem is that, by the time these images and narratives have been filtered through the beliefs and judgments of our adult minds, they can be a far cry from the original. A more effective approach is to use our imagination to travel back in time and 're-live' those experiences – to see what we once saw, to feel what we once felt and to respond as we once responded. This is a process that incorporates all our senses and faculties - to see, to hear, to smell, to feel, and to reflect on what once was – and at the deepest level, still is. It takes some time, but with a little practice, anyone can do it.

Yet, even then, something is missing. What we no longer have are the childhood friends with whom we shared and explored this world of mingled joy, anticipation, fear and make-believe. Of course, we could always invite our adult partners to participate in our regressions, and I have certainly learned much through this fascinating exercise. Conversely, why not create a relationship with an experienced expert on the subject of childhood and adolescence, one who actually lives and breathes in that realm? Such experts are all around, looking to us for connection and wanting, above all else, to be seen and heard.

This brings me to the enduring proposition that lies at the very heart of this book: *By reconnecting with ourselves through our relationships with our children, we will grow together, and together we can change the world.*

I realize this is a sweeping statement that most self-respecting researchers wouldn't touch at any price, but I have already amassed sufficient evidence to make it a hypothesis worthy of serious consideration. In countless relationships between parents and their children, and between professional helpers and their young clients, I have witnessed the profound changes that can occur on both sides when the authentic Self of one, is made available

> *By reconnecting with ourselves through our relationships with our children, we will grow together, and together we can change the world.*

to the Other. Whatever the skeptics might choose to believe, there is no loss of respect or confusion of roles and responsibilities on either side. In such encounters, adults are free to be who they are, children are free to be children and each is free to be curious about the other. Through this process, the bond of dependency is gradually transformed into a union between two unique human beings, moving in their own way along their own separate developmental pathways. This is what I mean when I say, "together we can change the world." As adults authentic expression always carries the risk of ridicule and rejection but for me, this seems like a relatively small price to pay for the liberation of the Self.

To bring this closer to home, I recall the precious hours I spent with my father shortly before he died. He spoke to me as never before; about his own poverty-stricken childhood, his hopes and aspirations as a young man, his love for my mother, his fears for himself and our family during the Second World War, and his dreams of the future for his two boys. He told me what it was like to be a father, *my* father, and how he and my mother had worried about my less than impressive school performances and the dissolution of my first marriage. He talked about death and his belief that "something keeps going after the body chucks in the towel." Then he listened as I told my own story; about growing up in our family, my world 'on the outside,' and my life with my partner Judith. He didn't say much but he didn't have to. The light that returned to his fading eyes, along with his thoughtful nods and occasional smiles, told me everything I wanted to know. This wasn't about communication; it was about communion. This world-weary old man loved me beyond words. On the long flight home, as I considered the prospect of never seeing him again, a brief surge of anger drifted into a heavy sadness. At the age of forty-two I had been offered an inside glimpse of the man who was my father, and I wanted more – much more. I spent the rest of the journey speculating about how both our lives might have been different if I'd had this information at the time when I most needed it. He died three months later.

My 'research' may fall short on acceptable empirical standards, but there is one conclusion I am prepared to stand by without further evidence: it isn't openness and authenticity that keeps us apart from one another, it's the defenses and deceptions we create to protect ourselves from being seen for who we really are. To qualify this conclusion,

I should point out that the adults in my 'non-randomized' sample all possessed a reasonably secure and contained sense of Self. They did not unload their own fragmentation and leave the child to pick up the pieces. As responsible teachers, they shared what they considered to be in the best interests of the child, and always in ways the child could understand. This requires sensitivity to the unique developmental history and needs of the child, along with a clear sense of where one Self ends and the Other begins. Authenticity is not the same as 'transparency,' and this must be fully understood by anyone who wishes to be in relationship with children.

It isn't openness and authenticity that keeps us apart from one another, it's the defenses and deceptions we create to protect ourselves from being seen for who we really are.

If we are to create a new kind of partnership with our children, one based upon mutual respect and curiosity, it is we, the adults, who must take the lead by being clear and honest about our hopes and expectations. I don't wish to prescribe what this should look like but, having spent over forty years working with troubled young people, I am prepared to throw out a few ideas about how we might start the ball rolling.

Relational Parenting

We might begin by eradicating, once and for all, the archaic belief that 'unquestioning obedience' is a legitimate parenting objective. We will always be their teachers, but the time has come for us to focus on teaching our children how to learn, rather than what to learn. Their future now depends upon their ability to create new visions and opportunities and, for this, we need to foster their curiosity and nurture their belief in themselves as creative, caring, conscious and responsible beings. The object of the exercise is for them to become responsible to themselves and not accountable to us.

In this cause, we must learn how to acknowledge and set them free from our own misplaced agendas. As caring parents, we all want the best for our kids, but we cannot hold them responsible for realizing our own unfulfilled dreams and aspirations – that's our job. As loving parents, we want our children to love us in return, but love is not a commodity to be traded according to some unspoken behavioral contract. For young children, love is about being looked after. The words "I love you Mommy" may be re-assuring, but they are essentially a learned response to parental expectations. For older kids, love is about hanging in when the going gets tough, as it always will be. The love we are all seeking only becomes truly reciprocal when it's experienced and expressed unconditionally. This is the love that becomes possible only as the authentic Self becomes known. It is love the Self needs to move toward wholeness. If we do our own work, we may be able to offer this love to our children, but let's stop kidding ourselves; we cannot get this from them. If we hang onto this belief, we will continue to regard them as 'failures,' and they will respond accordingly.

The time has come for us to focus on teaching our children how to learn, rather than what to learn. … The object of the exercise is for them to become responsible to themselves and not accountable to us.

To consider children as our partners in the exploration and expression of life, we might also need to re-examine our attitude toward the phase of life we refer to as "childhood." Since we have chosen to remain detached from our own kids, the term has acquired most of the characteristics of a diagnostic category. Such a classification might be defined thus: *Childhood is an incomplete and diminished state of being that, given normal conditions and a reasonable amount of care and attention, will naturally pass through specific developmental phases before the symptoms subside and adulthood is attained. In most cases, the individual (child) will eventually adapt to the familial and cultural norms with only transitory difficulties. Should the symptoms appear to persist beyond any specified phase, this might be indicative of an underlying pathology and professional advice should be sought immediately. Treatment for the condition of childhood may involve some psychological intervention but nowadays most symptoms can be cleared up quickly with an ever-increasing range of drugs. These should be administered only under the supervision of a duly qualified professional.*

Of course, this last passage is something of a spoof, but it reflects an attitude that is not uncommon among those who should know better. More seriously, it also contains a fundamental fallacy that can be found in most of the classifications listed in the psychiatric diagnostic manuals. I would like to suggest that there is no such thing as 'childhood' as we have come to understand it. What we have here is an arbitrary clustering of variables that can be found in all of us and, like all stereotypes, it refers to nothing that actually exists. When it comes to childhood, not even 'age' can be cited as a necessary condition. As someone once said, if you scratch the surface of a sixty-year-old man, you will find a five-year-old boy. I have waited sixty years to test this hypothesis and can now say that I find it overwhelmingly supported by the evidence.

Given the stance I have taken, I'm not about to reel off a list of nifty new answers to the old worn-out questions. I believe the time has come for us to go back to the original source of our knowledge and generate new questions from a much broader and more exciting range of interests. To this end, I'm suggesting that we look again at this period we call "childhood" in much the same way as a child might explore some aspect of the world for the first time; with wide-eyed wonder and unfettered curiosity. As adults, our natural tendency is to look outside for such information, but I am convinced that the acquisition of knowledge begins and ends with our own experience, and that this is as close as we will ever come to the "truth".

This experiential approach does not imply that our enquiry is destined to be either undisciplined or unscientific. Reviewing new information and testing this against what we already 'know' is the essence of scientific methodology. When we are grounded in the knowledge of our own experience, we can listen carefully to what the 'experts' have to say without abandoning ourselves to their wisdom, however brilliant it might seem. Alternatively if we sacrifice our Self on the altar of abstract learning, we have nothing of substance to share with other Selves. Unfortunately this detached and depersonalized approach to learning is widely considered to be the only way to go, and we call it "education". So when we educate our children this way, we deprive them of the most powerful learning experience – the opportunity to learn through direct contact with another caring, sharing and nurturing human being.

Given the opportunity, children will always help us to see our Selves more clearly. Free from the pretenses and distortions of the demanding ego, the mirror they offer reflects the essence and the innocence of our core humanness.

On the other side of the equation, to talk about children as our 'teachers' is a well-worn cliché, but they are, and function as a teacher in a most exquisite way. Given the opportunity and trust, they will share their 'truth' without censorship. They tell us what is immediate and important, and they are always there whenever we are ready to listen. By contrast, we adults are inclined to strategically deny or disguise our 'truth'. We hide behind the pretentious belief that what we say should never be challenged and that our children should conform to our beliefs and expectations. My point is that, given the opportunity, children will always help us to see our Selves more clearly. Free from the pretenses and distortions of the demanding ego, the mirror they offer reflects the essence and the innocence of our core humanness. To listen to a child with no other agenda than to hear and understand is to know again what we have chosen to forget. And whatever we see, let us not forget there is no fundamental division between them and us. From womb to tomb, we are all human beings stumbling along our own unique developmental pathway, sharing time together, while attending to our own particular experiences and aspirations. Though our responsibilities and obligations might be very different at any point in time, there is always something to be learned from the sharing of that experience.

Some Personal Memories of Home

If you are finding it difficult to take all this at face value, I can certainly empathize. Not only do these ideas stand in sharp contrast to my own memories of childhood, they also challenge pretty well everything I was taught as a professional. For reasons I never fully understood, and nobody ever questioned, I always knew I wanted to work with children. Significant others nodded their approval and applauded my good intentions, but whatever motivated me in the first place, remained a mystery. Sometimes, in sheer frustration, I would ask myself why the hell I was doing this, rather than pursuing my thespian dreams. Yet I continued on the same career pathway, rarely looking back, and only occasionally looking forward.

In a sense, my whole life has been a mystery of my own creation. The more I tried to figure it out, the more confusing it became, and the further I seemed to be from the 'truth'. The questions I asked were the same questions I asked as a child, but as a child the answers were simple and satisfying, wrought from direct experience. Later they became tricky and trivial, searching for a place in a complex matrix of ideas. As a child, I lived in a real world where every moment had a secret waiting to unfold. It was full of excitement and fear. But, as I invested more and more time thinking my way through life, my head grew tired of its creations and something in my belly yearned for the good old days.

I'm not saying this from 'memory' in the traditional sense of the word, but from the feelings and sensations that still sweep over me whenever I wander aimlessly back down the dimly lit alleyways that led me into adulthood. Sometimes, when my mind ceases its incessant chatter and settles into some quiet corner, these feelings find their own way into places long since forgotten or for whatever reason, dismissed. Suddenly I am there again, not in my mind or my imagination, but really there. Sometimes the images are clear and vivid and sometimes vague, like the shadows lurking on the basement wall, but there I am in the middle of it all, startlingly aware, fully in the moment, tenaciously curious and wonderfully alive.

So, what happened? Why is my mind so set to stifle the excitement and spontaneity I once cherished? Why does it still urge me to "grow up" and "be quiet", whenever I try to free myself from its neatly packaged reality? Is this some form of developmental imperative, or is it simply because my mind, so curious one moment and so dismissive the next, is now committed to another place; an external adult world of infinite ideas and relentless expectations? Is it possible that I am caught between two incompatible realities, one on the inside that tells me who I am, and one on the outside telling me who I should be and what I should do? And is my mind really committed to preserving one at the expense of the other?

But, regardless of what Freud, or anybody else, has said, what if there is no such division, other than that which my mind has created for its own purposes? What if these two alienated realities were to speak to one another? Could I then reclaim the magic of my disenfranchised past, or would it simply provide more grist for my mind to grind into yet another batch of cerebral corn bread? As one mindful person once observed, when the mind asks itself a question and then goes off in search of the answer, there is an immediate conflict of interest.

Well, the fact that I'm able to ask such questions suggests that my mind is indeed capable of embracing both realities. All I have to do is urge it in that direction. Yet, this implies that I am more than my mind, that I can inhabit both realms without being contained by either. So who, or what, am I? Am I the creator of these things? If so, is there any limit to my creative abilities, or can I construct my own life in whatever way I choose? With stuff like this to sort out, chances are my life will continue to be a mystery - thank God.

What I do know is, at some point in my life, the focus of the mystery changed. I remained incurably curious, but more about the unknown world "out there" than the world I had come to know on the inside. For some reason I gave up the unbridled enthusiasm of my childhood to find a place for my Self in a world inhabited by others. Out there, among their demands and expectations, the familiar and enchanted place that was my home seemed hopelessly inadequate and unacceptable. There was a time when I continued to invite people in, but one by one, they drifted away until, eventually, nobody

Is it possible that I am caught between two incompatible realities, one on the inside that tells me who I am, and one on the outside telling me who I should be and what I should do?

came, and to my mind, nobody cared. Occasionally I would open the door, but those who stopped to look in, even those who had once accepted my hospitality, would snigger and walk away. I felt ashamed and wondered what it would be like to spend the rest of my life locked in my room alone. Finally, I made the decision to leave, and stepped tentatively outside, slowly closing the door behind me.

I was scared – no, *terrified* - and promised myself I would always return home if things got rough. But I never did. Gradually, I carved out a niche for myself along the main highway, traveling first on foot, then by bike, then by bus and then by car, taking my place in the steady stream of traffic toward imaginary destinations. And along the way, I created new resting-places, each one grander than the one before. However much I tried, I never could find my way back to that magic place in Nowhere.

But my search has not been entirely in vain. Forcing my curiosity inwards, I began to find bits and pieces of my lost life stuffed under the cushions, hidden behind the furniture and crammed behind the walls of my paper castles. I became an avid collector of my own remnants, always looking for that missing piece and dreaming of the day when I could finally complete the set and put it all back together where it used to be - at the center of my life. Somehow, I seemed to be carrying the pieces with me wherever I went, although I also had this sense that it was only my mind that dismantled my childhood haven and buried the memory within its darkest reaches. And this is why it remains so aloof and dismissive whenever I sneak away and allow my secrets to come flooding back, from the inside out.

Now in my mid-sixties, I continue to be surprised by what I find behind the complex array of obstacles and deceptions I have carefully and strategically placed between my Self and the world. On reflection, however, I usually find that the 'surprise' is not so much a discovery of something new as a re-discovery of something lost. Trying to understand why I chose to create these hiding places in the first place has made it possible for me to take a kinder and more loving attitude toward my Self, and toward those from whom I once sought protection. The real excitement comes whenever I take the risk to set these secrets free - to allow the world I discover on the inside to spill out into the world I have come to know on the outside. Whenever this happens, I feel a familiar trembling, a sense of uncertainty that I once thought of as fear. Now I think of it as "aliveness". Sometimes, when my secrets are met with warmth and acceptance, it's as if my life is transformed into a single entity: an ecstatic blend of innocence, freedom and relatedness that converges into an overwhelming sense of being in the world. I can compare it only with those rare and wonderful moments in my childhood when I felt truly seen, heard and accepted by someone I cared about. Now, as an adult, I know enough to seek out people who are willing to share my curiosity, to bring their Selves and their own secrets into the world and meet me somewhere in the middle. I call this a *meeting of Selves*.

The Professional Pathway

Before concluding this chapter, I'd like to share a few details of my professional career. This is not an exercise in self-indulgence, but rather a sincere desire for you to gain some understanding of how my beliefs and perspectives came to be. My hope is you will find some elements and themes that jibe with your own experience.

As I look back over my 65 years of messing about on this planet, it's hard to believe I've spent so much of my life working with troubled kids. My earliest childhood fantasies and schoolboy dreams gave no hint things would turn out this way. So often I set off in other directions, but such diversions were always short-lived and for the most part, unremarkable. There was a time when I would have attributed my lack of purpose to circumstances beyond my control, but over the years, I've slowly, though at times reluctantly, come to realize that all the significant choices have been mine. I think this is what growing up is all about.

Perhaps I never really had whatever it takes to become a welder, actor, writer, musician or secret agent, so I conveniently slipped back into something more available and do-able. Indeed, my early attempts to secure a regular pay cheque had all the characteristics of a drifter, motivated more by circumstance and opportunity than passion and purpose. I enjoyed trying on adult roles, sometimes real and sometimes imagined but, as the expectations and demands closed in, I would delight in breaking the rules before jumping into some alternative persona. Even in graduate school, I carefully avoided any decision that might cast me in some professional mold and the chairman of my Ph.D. dissertation committee became convinced that my apparent lack of commitment and responsibility reflected some unresolved problem of adolescence. Oddly enough, I was running a large residential treatment center for emotionally disturbed children at that time, and considered myself to be thoroughly committed to my work and acutely aware of my responsibilities.

I now believe my fear was that if I abandoned my own incomplete childhood in the service of becoming an adult, I would cut myself off from something far more valuable than any professional role or status could possibly offer. Much as I enjoyed reading about what Freud, Piaget and B.F. Skinner had to say, I was always more interested in knowing kids directly than learning *about* them through other's theories. And, while I worked diligently to develop my diagnostic and therapeutic skills, I still preferred doing things *with* kids rather than doing things *to* them.

Behind the pretensions and performances of my emerging professional identity, I always knew I could learn far more about young Jimmy Tasker in a twenty-minute chat before bedtime, than anything I could glean from reading the entire works of Sigmund Freud or sifting through the latest battery of psychometric tests. Theoretical models, diagnostic tools and intervention techniques were all very interesting, but these things did little to satisfy my inherent curiosity about what Jimmy's life was really like. The information I needed could only come from the lad himself, and my interpretations could only be drawn from the hazy recollections of my own childhood and adolescence. To enhance such understanding, I needed the freedom to bring these things together without being burdened by the belief that I had to change him, fix him or even teach him in some way. In other words, I needed to work toward a personal relationship that would bring both of us together, for our mutual benefit. Whenever I shared this belief with colleagues, or in graduate seminars, it was generally dismissed as being unprofessional, and I came to accept their position rather than risk the possibility of rejection, or even worse, academic failure.

The Kids in my Mirror

At some level, I understood there was something about the lives of kids that had profound relevance for my own life. Yet, like a good professional in the making, I turned my attention away from what they had to say about themselves and focused on what the experts had to say about them. In a sense, I abandoned my primary teachers, along with those precious gems of wisdom tossed out by kids when they're not concerned with giving adults what they believe adults want to hear. I forgot about seven year old Gordie Farrington who, when asked, "So what is it that lies deepest on inside Gordie?" put both hands on his belly and replied, "wieners and beans". I had little time to think about the indomitable Susie Marchand who, having demanded that the scary "Munsters" be exorcised from her bedroom, came down at eleven-o-clock one night in tears. "The Munsters are sad," she told us, "I can hear them crying outside. Please come up and tell them it's okay. They can share my room if they want, but they've gotta be quiet so I can get some fucking sleep." Then there was eleven-year-old Mike Richards who, after been repeatedly knocked to the ice in a hockey game finally turned to his assailant and screamed, "you shit-head, the only reason I hang around with you is because I thought you liked me."

But I did not forget about Mick Proctor, and I never will. Mick was a twelve-year-old slugger who had the misfortune to be in the first class I ever taught as a student teacher. He was unruly, undisciplined, uncontrollable and to all intents and purposes, un-teachable. It wasn't that I didn't like the tousle-headed monster. He had a clumsy charm about him, and his occasional wit belied his abysmal scholastic performance. But Mick pushed his luck far beyond what any rookie teacher might be expected to tolerate. In the staff room I complained to my tenured colleagues that Mick's behavior was disrupting the other kids in the class and their recommendation was unanimous – "the slipper".

These were the days, long before the advent of psychotropic medication, when corporal punishment was not only permitted but was the preferred strategy for subduing known terrorists and setting an example for any others that might be tempted by the forces of evil. In this particular school "the slipper" was an intrinsically benign object, usually an old gym shoe, housed in a cupboard beside the blackboard. But, in a more general and understood sense, the term referred to a ritual that, once initiated, had to be followed through with single-minded purpose and precision. While each teacher was granted some freedom to bring his or her own particular style to the occasion, the basic sequence of the procedure was bound firmly by consensus and tradition.

In short, the offender was either summoned or dragged to the front of the class. After a brief summary of the crime, the hostage was instructed to face the class and bend over. While in this pose, "the slipper" was taken from the cupboard, either by the teacher or, more dramatically, by another member of the class. This created an anticipatory delay, specifically designed to build emotional arousal, whether fear or excitement, among the spectators and participants. Then, at the moment of optimum intensity, the dedicated educator, slipper in hand, would spring into action, delivering a series of blows to the presented buttocks. The time invested in this segment of the ritual, and the number of blows delivered, were determined by the nature of the crime and the degree of dedication on the part of the deliverer. According to the formal prescription, the responses of the recipient should in no way serve to influence such decisions, but it was widely known that the failure to display any outward sign of distress would inevitably increase both the intensity and duration of the punishment. Then came the denouement; a period of quiet reflection before the class was allowed to return to its tedious routines.

I considered myself to be one of the new breeds – a rookie teacher determined not to perpetuate the barbarism of my own school days – and Mick quickly caught onto my mission. Resisting all attempts to divert him from his mischief, his disruptions in class escalated and his attitude toward me degenerated into the grossest levels of disrespect. My admonishments were met with a grin, and my demands rudely ignored. Sending him to "the office" was a waste of time since the Principal, a dedicated administrator, had made it perfectly clear that she considered discipline to be the responsibility of the classroom teacher. At first, his classmates were bemused by my unprecedented leniency, but gradually, this benign attitude began to turn into something more sinister as others began to 'try it on' with the new teacher. I was losing my place, my authority, in my classroom, and each day my energies became increasingly directed toward handling Mick Proctor rather than my educational responsibilities. My colleagues knew all about it and their whispered asides in the staff room did nothing to bolster my wilting confidence.

Finally, I broke. Following a particularly obnoxious act of defiance, I stormed over to Procter's desk and dragged him to the front of the class. With one hand still clasped around his arm, I opened the cupboard door and grabbed the slipper with the other. He struggled to get free, but my anger was more than enough to out-muscle a writhing twelve-year old. Driving my forearm into the middle of his back, I crunched him over my desk and brought the slipper down with all my might on his stretched out rear end. Then, for good measure, I delivered another blow with equal ferocity. At this point my energy and commitment began to dissipate and, as I released the pressure on his back, he turned his face away from the class and toward me. He was grinning – not grimacing but *grinning*. My fury returned in an instant, and before my mind had any chance to catch up with my actions, I had him pinned back on the desk and the slipper was at it again, hell bent on wiping the smirk from his face.

I have no clear recollection of what actually happened immediately following my assault on Mick Proctor. What I do remember is leaving the school that afternoon in a state of complete fragmentation. I was too shaky to ride my motorbike, so I decided to leave it in the sheds and walk home. As I passed groups of kids hanging around the playground and straggling along the streets, I tried to pick out the figure of Mick, but he was nowhere to be seen. Outside the classroom he was a loner who lived with his mother and elder brother in one of the old condemned houses by Welton canal. It was well known that his father was serving a lengthy prison sentence for countless offences, including aggravated assault. For reasons beyond my comprehension at the time, I diverted my journey home and made my way down the alleyways leading to the canal. I didn't know exactly where young Proctor lived, but there were only three adjoining row houses clustered together between two disused warehouses. The others had all been demolished.

Then I saw him. He was standing by the edge of the canal trying to coax a bedraggled looking dog to retrieve the sticks he was tossing into the water. He also saw me, but true to form, paid no heed to my approaching presence. "Where's your Ma?" I asked. "How should I know?" he muttered, "Where's yours?" It was a fair question but in the interests of making contact, I chose not to answer. "Doesn't look like that dog's going to go for it," I said as the creature wandered off to relieve itself on a mooring post. Without even glancing in my direction, the lad turned and walked away from me and toward the uncooperative animal. "Guess I'd better get meself a slipper," he said, to nobody in particular.

When I finally got home that evening, I couldn't tell you all that was churning in my mind. What I can tell you is that I sat in my chair with an unopened book on my lap and wept.

Like most kids, I learned very early in life that pleasing my parents and attending to the wishes of my teachers was the key to my survival, and I took this belief into the obligations of adulthood.

As it turns out, I came to know Mick Proctor quite well in the months that followed. I made a point of it. In some way I knew my relationship with him was important to both of us. Eventually, I also came to understand what prompted my behavior on that day and the source of the emotions that followed. As a teacher, I had become so attached to my role and the expectations it carried that I had little or no personal contact with the kids clustered together in that classroom. And the feelings that continued to haunt me did not spring from a sense of guilt and remorse, as I first suspected. These were the deep and unforgiving feelings of shame – a knowing that I had turned away from what I cherished above all things, the essence of my own humanity. My professional life would never be the same and, needless to say, I have never, and will never, strike out at a child again.

Hanging in and Burning out

Shame was not the only the personal matter to arise in my struggles to find a suitable professional label for my work. Throughout my early career, I fought to constrain a gnawing sense that that my life was not of my own making; that I was dancing to someone else's tune. Like most kids, I learned very early in life that pleasing my parents and attending to the wishes of my teachers was the key to my survival, and I took this belief into the obligations of adulthood. When the weight of these expectations became overwhelming, I resorted to token acts of resistance, but these occasional flights of fancy aroused little interest amongst those I most wanted to please and produced no sustained satisfaction for myself.

The truth is that my compelling need to please others had become my own deeply rooted agenda, regardless of the circumstances, and my bouts of rebellion were more against me than anyone else. Without my overriding need for approval, my adolescence may not have been delayed, and it's quite likely these episodes would have been ugly enough to have me labeled and subjected to some form of professional intervention. I mention this because the troubles of so many of the youngsters who have come to my attention over the years, began with their bungled attempts to break from the agendas of their parents and prove to themselves and the world that they could take charge of their own lives.

So there was I, flitting from one professional role to another, trying to fix other people's lives in the vain hope that I could please everybody along the way. As any rational mind should know, this is a task doomed for failure – you can no more fix people's lives than you can make them happy - but people like me continue to try, to the point of exhaustion and despair. In my subsequent work with 'burned-out' professional helpers, I saw this same theme emerging time and time again. Rather than recognize the futility of their quest, so many of these otherwise intelligent men and women chose to up the ante by increasing their commitment to education and training, while scrambling for the latest fad in the seductive boutique of nifty techniques and intervention strategies. Some rose high enough in the professional ranks to settle for social status as a measure of their success. Others kept their illusions alive by buying into their own professional mystique. Over time, many found themselves unable to ward off the debilitating cluster of symptoms that came to be known as 'burn-out'.

And I was one of them.

The term 'burn-out' is really no different from all those other labels we in the mental health business like to slap

The gradual shift toward becoming the author in my own life has fundamentally changed my way of being in the world.

on the misery of people's lives. All are simplistic external judgments that purport to identify or explain complex internal experiences. Suffice to say that the genesis of my own misery is clearly outlined in the preceding paragraphs. Had it not been for the ultimatums laid down by my long-suffering partner, I might have languished in this state for years, but with my most cherished relationship on the line, I stumbled out on the trip people now call 'self-discovery,' but in my case, it was more like 'self-recovery'.

For me, this has been a long and arduous process that, I'm pleased to report, continues to this day. In that first transformational year, I not only confronted my addiction to pleasing others, but also uncovered the stunning irony that working with kids was something I wanted to do *for myself* and not merely for the approval of others, real or imagined. But awareness is not change - it's only an opportunity to explore possibilities. Placing my Self at the center of my life, making my own choices and holding myself responsible for the outcomes, became a moment-by-moment challenge and there have been many lapses along the way. Even now, when doubts arise, I catch myself looking to the outside for validation, or blaming others for my discontent. The recognition is not in my head but in my belly – the kind of hollowness I used to feel when childhood friends moved away, as they so often did. And, to this day, I still enjoy the approval and appreciation of others, although I am now more likely to take these offerings back to the scrutiny of my own evaluations.

However simple and obvious this might appear, the gradual shift toward becoming the author in my own life has fundamentally changed my way of being in the world. When I take full ownership of my own experiences, I am able to express my thoughts and feelings without fear of rejection or retribution, while remaining open to the thoughts and feelings of others. The old urge to please and fix is still around, but when I am able to see this as a reflection of my own needs, I can step in before too much damage is done. Free from the burden of taking responsibility for the experiences and actions of others, I can simply allow myself to be there, and invite others to join me in something called a relationship. In bringing this into my work, I have often found myself confronted by both clients and colleagues who believed that I was abandoning my professional responsibilities and obligations. Yet, within my own experience, I had come to know that my attempts to fix other people's lives were a lost cause in the service of my own ego and a debilitating imposition on my fellow human beings.

I still don't fully understand why as a professional, it took me so long to rediscover my simple curiosity about the mystery of my client's lives. Throughout the early years of my career as a therapist I went to great lengths to replace such fascinating ambiguity with diagnostic certainty. My training in clinical psychology offered the false assurance that I could be the 'knower with the knowledge,' and that the only mystery to be solved was where my clients might fit into my theoretical framework and what I needed to do to treat their problems. In relating to my clients, my task was to remain objective. This meant that I should discount the emotional content and remain focused on the 'real' problem. In order to do this, it was essential that my own personal feelings should be similarly discounted and at all costs, kept out of the equation.

With the best of intentions, I was a diligent and dedicated therapist, using my knowledge and skills to make things better for others and in some small way, to make the world a better place. Now I find it hard to believe

I actually harbored such delusions of grandeur. In my enthusiasm, I failed to understand that a more caring and compassionate world can only be created through guileless human contact and shared intentions. Determined to make things happen, I would volunteer to take on the most difficult and resistant clients, reading more and more about psychopathology and taking countless courses and workshops to improve my therapeutic techniques. The greater the challenge, the more I applied myself to the task, often resenting my clients for their failure to respond to my efforts. There was even a time when I became envious of my psychiatric colleagues who could always reach for the medication when things ground to a halt. It's hardly surprising that I made myself sick.

Through my long and turbulent period of recovery, I began to realize that I'd been the one doing all the work. My perspective from the *outside in* would have it no other way, since it was my knowledge, my skill and my personal resources that were needed to initiate and sustain the enterprise. To hold my clients in any way responsible would be to blame them for their difficulties. Yet, in the most profound way, they are responsible, or more precisely, response-able. To deny this is to turn them into victims – casualties of forces beyond their control and lacking the resources for change. Given my inherent need to make people happy, combined with my years of training and practice in the field, it's understandable I would slip easily into the victim mentality and that I would take the same stance toward myself when I became debilitated by the experience known as "burn-out". I took some time off work, followed all the usual prescriptions and would have returned to do it all over again had it not been for three of my more enlightened teachers; Bennet Wong, Jock Mckeen and Will Schutz. These individuals urged me to examine how my condition was the outcome of choices I had made, with or without awareness.

The idea that we humans are constantly making choices, either consciously or unconsciously, may not sit well with the clockwork scientists and among those who find solace in the victim mentality. But, if any growth or change is to take place within the human condition (individually or collectively), we must learn how to become aware of the choices we make and take responsibility for the outcomes. As the popular writer Shad Helmstetter has suggested: "If you'd like to know what your choices have been, look at yourself and the life you have lived. What you see is the choices you've made." (p. 123) However much we might find ourselves restricted by circumstances or overwhelmed by feelings of helplessness, our range of options is always limitless. This applies to the man who stands on the gallows with a noose around his neck as much as it applies to the wealthy widow in Macey's Department Store. The nature of the human mind is such that our options are not presented from the outside - they are created from the inside.

> *If any growth or change is to take place within the human condition (individually or collectively), we must learn how to become aware of the choices we make and take responsibility for the outcomes.*

Within the broader context, the matter of choice becomes considerably more complex and I will discuss the issue in more detail later. Let me make it clear that I do not believe a woman killed by a sniper's bullet in a shopping mall is responsible for her own tragedy. Nor would I argue that children in Somalia have chosen a pathway of disease and starvation. My point is only that we all have the ability to influence and respond to the external world in infinite ways – not that we each have the power to change external conditions whenever they are not to our liking. To fall back on a well-worn cliché, it's not what happens to us that determines our freedom; it's how we respond to what happens.

Our ability to examine our options and create new opportunities is the resource we now need if we are to take that next developmental step. If the decisions we make reflect the fullness of our Selves as caring, compassionate and responsible agents, then the quality of our lives on this planet can only be enhanced. On the other hand, if we *choose* to ignore this potential, abandon our Selves to the cosmos and do nothing on our own behalf our destiny will be determined solely by external forces. I know many thinking people who believe the universe will take care of us in some mystical way, but I have little or no evidence to support this hypothesis. My own belief is that the universe is indifferent to our well being, and evidence clearly suggests that our planet has had enough of our irresponsibility. I realize I cannot provide conclusive proof for my belief either but, faced with both propositions, I prefer to live with the assumption that I have the ability to choose. To defer once more to the words of Shad Helmstetter: "If you were given only one choice – to choose or not to choose – which would *you* choose?" (p.53)

It's not what happens to us that determines our freedom; it's how we respond to what happens.

This is a difficult notion to sustain, particularly if you happen to work with young people who've been abused or whose needs have been grossly neglected. I still react with anger and sadness when I consider the histories of these children, but there can be no changing what has occurred in the past. That was then and this is now. My empathy and understanding is essential but, sooner or later, it is they who must examine the choices they have made, and the alternatives they are capable of creating on their own behalf. Of course, I realize that dependent infants and children don't have the freedom or experience to make adult choices, but I can think of no more important task for a parent or teacher than assisting and supporting them to expand those options and make responsible decisions for themselves.

As a professional, my challenge is to work toward the kind of relationships in which all of this can take place. In this regard, the traditional therapist-client relationship, with its prescriptions and cures, is not only counter-productive - it's potentially toxic. Physical disabilities aside, I have come to the conclusion that all our developmental interruptions were created in relationships and can only be resolved in relationships. Children whose basic needs have not been met cannot move toward higher levels of personal decision-making and self-responsibility unless these needs are recognized and addressed within the context of a warm, caring and responsive relationship. Only through such relationships will they develop the trust to bring their protected Selves forward. Only when that Self shows up will they begin to make self-responsible choices. Simply stated, my job is to be there, to welcome that young person's Self into the world, and offer the support he or she will need to stay connected. If I am not fully present, or if I choose to hide behind some professional facade, the child's fledgling Self will remain unseen, unheard, and alone. For anything of value to take place between us, I too must show up, ready to convene a meeting of Selves. My ability and willingness to do this is *my* work.

What I'm suggesting demands the highest levels of professional skill and personal commitment on the part of the practitioner. At the same time, it's an act of faith – a fundamental belief that all of us, children and adults, possess all the inner resources we need to move on and create the life we want in our own way. As a professional, I cannot presume to know and understand the inner life of my clients, but my curiosity serves as a constant invitation for self-exploration on both sides. In effect, the more I am able to understand my client's experience, the more I am able to understand my own. Nor can I presume to diagnose their problems or come up with the answers. What I can do is to bring myself into a relationship, along with whatever education, training and experience I've managed to pick up along the way. In the final analysis, I know it is they who must do the bulk of the work, and it is they who must take responsibility for whatever decisions they choose to make. I cannot claim success for such outcomes, nor am I about to take responsibility when things fall apart. I can rejoice in their accomplishments and share my sadness in their despair. But my only real responsibility is to my Self – to work to the best of my ability, to remain open and curious, to keep my client's best interest in mind and to retain my own sense of personal integrity in the process.

CHAPTER TWO

The New Science of the Self

The story of your life does not begin at birth, or even at the moment of conception. The drama of human life has been unfolding on this planet for a very long time, and the legacy of that history is bestowed upon all of us from the outset, regardless of our particular location and circumstances. Nor does your story conclude with your final breath. Whatever you have created, whether judged to be miraculous or mundane, shimmering or shameful, will be forever etched into the collective consciousness of the universal order. This is the consciousness that makes us distinctly human and connects us to all human experience, past, present and future. Whether we like it or not, we will always remain an integral part of the whole.

If you agree with this statement, I invite you to read on and live your life accordingly. If you are unsure, or strongly disagree, at least allow me to state my case.

The idea that human consciousness is a bona fide ingredient in the cosmic casserole has been around a long time. In the Western world it was beautifully explicated by psychoanalyst Carl Jung and given the scientific seal of approval by Albert Einstein. More recently, the proposition that consciousness is as real as matter has found a solid location in the science of the 'New Physics'.

In order to dialogue with those who claim to be informed, we need to match their knowledge with our own curiosity.

Drawing from a sweeping re-examination of the subatomic realm, physicists are now presenting us with a radically different picture of how the universe works. Perhaps the most dramatic feature of this analysis is the 'discovery' that each element contains a duality of functions – particle and wave - giving rise to complex energy systems that do not conform to our standard view of cause and effect predictability. Extrapolations of these principles can now be found in many forms, including the formulations of 'Chaos Theory' described by James Gleick in 1988.

This isn't easy stuff for most of us to comprehend, but if collective awareness is essential for purposeful collective action, then understand it we must. If we are to take the next step along the developmental continuum, we can no longer afford to allow our view of ourselves and the universe to be handed down by 'experts' and soothsayers, however brilliant or enlightened we deem them to be. If they have something to tell us, then it needs to be expressed in ways we can all understand. If they cannot, or will not, communicate their insights in this way, we have no reason to take them seriously. On the other side, we will not move beyond our collective adolescence until we decide to become active seekers of information rather than passive recipients. In order to dialogue with those who claim to be informed, we need to match their knowledge with our own curiosity. In order to grasp the simple truth, we need to understand the complexity from which it emerges. If we can talk to a computer salesperson about hard drives and megabytes, we should also be able to talk to a scientist about Bose-Einstein condensates. This doesn't mean we should all aspire to be physicists or biologists, only that we learn how to communicate, interpret whatever they have to say, and draw our own conclusions.

Without such a commitment, the chances are we will continue to latch onto the most simplistic interpretations and turn them into some kind of magic. A classic example is the current fascination with 'Attraction Theory'. Crudely extracted from principles of subatomic processes, the purveyors of this fad would have you believe that if you really concentrate on what you really want, you will attract whatever this might be and the universe will do the rest. Presumably this is more reliable than prayer since the universe is less demanding than God and moves in less mysterious ways. As always, wherever there are suckers to be found, there's money to be made. Marketed as "The Secret," the popularity of this exercise in magical or wishful thinking is a disturbing reflection of our arrested developmental state. The irony is that many of those who buy into such fanciful and unfounded beliefs consider themselves to be progressive (and even enlightened) 'thinkers'.

> *Becoming aware of our place in the scheme of things is no less challenging than becoming aware of our internal experiences.*

Becoming aware of our place in the scheme of things is no less challenging than becoming aware of our internal experiences. Both require the same level of curiosity, commitment and discipline. Developmental shifts occur when these two perspectives become integrated within a unified state of 'knowing'. Even then, since awareness is defined as a state of openness, such knowledge can only be held until further notice, subject to new information from either domain. When it comes to understanding the fascinating new images of 'reality' revealed through the quantum lens, our willingness to meet such a challenge may well turn out to be a critical factor in determining the future of our place on the planet. My own struggle to decipher even the most fundamental shapes and shadows is ongoing. Once I manage to get past the unfamiliar language to grasp the underlying concepts, my mind then balks at the prospect of confronting my most basic life-long assumptions and beliefs. For anyone setting out on this trail, I recommend two books that have sustained my curiosity and helped me to gain some glimmer of understanding.

In my view, David Bohm's classic work, *Wholeness and the Implicate Order*, published in 1980, is still a brilliant introduction to quantum theory. This is a scholarly text, but with a little effort and some re-reading, the substance and significance of what Bohm has to say are readily available to the committed reader. In 1990, Dianah Zohar extrapolated the insights of Bohm's thesis into the realm of everyday life, specifically the arena of human relationships, with her book *The Quantum Self*. Particularly pertinent to my statement at the beginning of this chapter, she writes: "Through the process of quantum memory, each of us carries within himself, woven into the fabric of his own soul, all the intimate relationships he has ever had, just as each of us weaves into his being all of his other interactions with the outside world." In the following paragraph, she goes on to say: "Intimate relationship itself is accounted for in quantum terms by the overlapping of one person's wave function with that of another. The quality and dynamics of that relationship, however, depend on the many variables that can affect any wave system" (p.137). With reference to our inherent ability to take conscious action on our own behalf, Zohar notes: "In quantum terms, however, it is impossible to define our human being without confronting the meaning of freedom. Consciousness, by its very nature as a quantum system, is a thread of freedom running through our lives at every moment" (italics mine) (p.177).

These two books may seem a little outdated, since much has been written about the quantum perspective over the last decade. I recommend them because they both take the reader through the presenting complexity of the phenomena as a means to understanding the simple 'truths' that lie beyond. We may not know too much about how global consciousness actually works at this point, although we can all run around screaming that something has to be done about global warming. Yet I believe these phenomena are inextricably linked, and in the long run, our survival depends more on understanding the former than solving the latter. But we don't have the time to run endless laboratory tests, collect the necessary data and establish the mathematical proofs. This isn't the realm of science in the traditional sense - it's the stuff of the human mind. The question is, once we become aware of our collective consciousness, can we become purposeful and creative in the contributions we make to preserving and enriching our lives on this planet? The answer to this question is embedded in our developmental history.

As with all forms of life, our earliest challenge is to learn how to survive in this strange, and potentially hazardous place. Thankfully, nature usually plays its part in helping to ensure our most basic needs are met and that we are biologically capable of adapting to the physical world. Unlike most other life forms on this planet, surviving and adapting to our immediate circumstances is not the object of the exercise; it's only the prelude. Our lives are not simply the product of our genetic and biological pre-dispositions interacting with external forces. For centuries, historians have been documenting our ability to shape our external environments to suit our own purposes. Through the discipline of psychology, we have become increasingly aware of how we use our conscious minds to create the substance and meaning of our lives on the inside. Now, scientists are placing us at the very center of the creative cycle by showing how we are constantly modifying our biological make-up through our thoughts, beliefs and actions – even to the level of DNA. In other words, we are speaking to our bodies and our bodies are listening and responding. When body and mind respond to a single voice, they become one, and whatever is spoken from that place of unity is as close as we will ever come to the truth.

> *We are constantly modifying our biological make-up through our thoughts, beliefs and actions – even to the level of DNA.*

Of particular interest is the work of cell biologist Bruce Lipton. In his book *The Biology of Belief,* published in 2005, he describes how each individual human cell responds to its environment by adopting one of two distinctive modalities – growth and closure. Growth occurs when the organism remains open to environmental stimuli, but when such influences present a perceived threat, the system shuts down for its own protection. It is impossible for these two modalities to be operating at the same time. In multi-cellular systems, such as the human body, each individual cell is actively engaged in either one modality or the other. The more the organism senses an external threat, the greater the percentage of cells involved in the protective mode. This inhibition of growth cuts off the creation of life-sustaining energy that, in the extreme case, may cause the entire system to close down – a condition Lipton refers to as being "scared to death."

The psychological implications are readily apparent. If we live our lives in fear, our vitality, creativity and innate potential will be proportionately compromised. However, unlike other life forms, we humans possess a conscious mind that is capable of mediating between environmental conditions and internal experiences. In other words, we have the inherent ability to moderate even our most instinctual fears and organize our behavioral responses accordingly. By the same token, we are also capable of creating infinite fears and conjuring up spooks causing both body and mind to withdraw from the action. In short, we are the creators of both our ecstasy and our terror.

Within the same general framework, research biophysicist Candace Pert presents an impressive array of biological evidence to show how we are also the creators of our feelings and emotions. In her startling biographical work, *Molecules of Emotion*, this eminent scientist takes the notion of body-mind connection out of the realm of speculation and places it firmly within an established scientific paradigm. With regard to our unexplored freedom she writes: "Although the capacity for learning is to some extent present in even the simplest creature, will power is the uniquely human 'ghost in the machine'..." (p. 135).

This is by no means a new idea among philosophers, but Western science has traditionally shied away from anything that appears to invest the human organism with free will. In presenting their findings, scientists like Lipton and Pert place themselves among a growing number of researchers who are deconstructing the old beliefs and re-connecting the abstractions of science with the wisdom of human intuition and insight. My hope is that other pioneers of the 'New Science' will follow their example and

If we live our lives in fear, our vitality, creativity and innate potential will be proportionately compromised ... we are also capable of creating infinite fears and conjuring up spooks causing both body and mind to withdraw from the action... we are the creators of both our ecstasy and our terror.

Contrary to the popular adage that 'our children are our future,' I am firmly convinced that their future now rests in our hands as never before.

find ways to communicate their discoveries with all who are prepared to listen.

The overall message is clear. We are indeed at the centre of our lives with the inherent ability to influence our external and internal environments in infinite ways. Perhaps we can now put the tedious old 'nature versus nurture' debate to rest and get on with the task at hand. Whether this represents a relatively recent phase in our evolution, or is simply an affirmation of what has always been, is a matter for the scientists and historians to mull over. My pragmatic stance is that we have what it takes to transform our lives and reshape our world - in that order. This is a reversal of how we have managed our affairs up to this point, but I believe adopting an 'inside-out' strategy is the first step in breaking free from the shackles of our collective adolescence. And, as I argued in the preceding chapter, it is we the adults, who must take this critical shift. Contrary to the popular adage that 'our children are our future,' I am firmly convinced that their future now rests in our hands as never before. It may be too late to change what we are leaving behind, but at least we can help them to discover the resources they will need to shape their own destinies.

First we need to acknowledge that the old ways are redundant and have become counter productive. There's no point in teaching kids how to succeed in a world that is glaringly unsustainable. However much we may want them to become engineers, professional golfers, or lawyers, we need to recognize these desires as our own misplaced agenda and focus our attention on their ability to make choices on their own behalf. Our primary concern is not with their achievements, past, present or future, but with the day-to-day aliveness and purpose that comes with the development of the Self. This isn't simply a matter of changing our parenting methods or teaching practices. If we are unsure or confused about our own sense of Self and its potentials, we are in no position to provide the guidance and support to the emerging Self of a child. In addition, if we are unable to make a clear distinction between our own needs and the developmental needs of the child, we will never grant the freedom necessary for that Self to grow and express its own volition; we cannot give to our children what we don't have for ourselves.

But we cannot expect our kids to sit quietly in their rooms while

Our attention actually changes the nature of the phenomena under observation. From this perspective, I would suggest that when we begin to see children as our partners in learning, we create the possibility of transforming bondage into bonding, to generate power with them rather than exercise power over them.

we get our act together. If they are to accept the challenge of moving our species into its next developmental phase, they need to be learning as we learn – not through coercion, but by invitation. Our renewed curiosity should match theirs, our respective discoveries shared and acknowledged. In the most fundamental sense, we need to engage them as our partners in learning. If we begin by seeing our children this way, we open the door to countless unexplored opportunities. To borrow a statement from the popular guru, Wayne Dyer, when we change the way we look at things, the things we look at change. This isn't simply a matter of selective perception and interpretation. One of the most remarkable tenets of quantum physics is that our attention actually changes the nature of the phenomena under observation. From this perspective, I would suggest that when we begin to see children as our partners in learning, we create the possibility of transforming bondage into bonding, to generate power with them rather than exercise power over them.

From the outset, we need to come to terms with what we already know. It's time to stop distorting the truth of our lives with opiates, drugs and illusions. Our feelings of anxiety, depression and despair are not demons to be eradicated; they are the stifled cries of the repressed Spirit. If we refuse to listen to our own voice, how will we be able to listen to the voices our children? If we declare ourselves to be incapable of acting on our own behalf, what could they possibly learn from our helplessness? Our only option is to pass on the illusion that some external force will eventually come along and make everything right. Some might call this "faith", but given the current state of life on our planet, I consider this to be a disastrous cop out. Listening and responding to our truth is an act of courage that can only be taken by one person at a time. This means you and me, and the guy who sells vegetables at the Saturday market. Together, we have ravished and squandered the resources of our planet. Now, when we call upon our Gods for our salvation, we insult all that is sacred and divine; when we begrudgingly bend to the exhortations of the environmentalists, we act as adolescents who have been told to clean up their rooms or find somewhere else to live.

My point is that our internal and external worlds mirror each other. Our planet is sick and depleted, as we are sick and depleted. If we continue to believe that the cure lies outside ourselves and choose to remain stuck in our inertia, we will lose our place as active participants in nature's purpose. Within the larger universal picture, our decision to opt out may not be that significant, but from the minute pixel of my life on beautiful Vancouver Island, it appears as a major tragedy, especially for our children. I find it hard to accept that we would come this far only to remain frozen on the brink of our most transformational developmental challenge – the shift from being mindless consumers of nature's resources to become conscious and legitimate contributors in its evolution. I am deeply saddened by the prospect of remaining unchanged, while watching our kids drift further into various states of meaninglessness, entitlement, confusion, resentment and rebellion. To me, this is even more disheartening than keeping track of the degradation caused by our unrelenting assaults on the planet.

I find it hard to accept that we would come this far only to remain frozen on the brink of our most transform-ational developmental challenge – the shift from being mindless consumers of nature's resources to become conscious and legit-imate contributors in its evolution.

Our urgent task is to turn our attention to our lives on the inside, moving through our fears and defenses to re-connect with the essence of our humanness. You may wish to think of this as Soul or Spirit - whatever the label, I'm convinced that the 'truth' of who we are, and where we fit into the scheme of things, is there waiting to be discovered. Whatever we discover serves to enlighten the whole. We can no longer afford to consider this as a quest reserved for the seekers, sages and mystics. Nor can we find our way through religious dogma, or by sitting quietly in church on Sunday. We must engage the Self directly in finding its own location in each of our lives. From this central, or sacred, place, the limitations we have chosen to impose upon our Selves can be critically examined and new choices made. Contrary to many, I don't believe that all we need to do is to reconnect with the universal source and surrender to the flow. Only when we recognize ourselves as conscious and purposeful beings can we begin to re-create the world in a way that supports our lives on this planet and affirms our inherent relatedness to the whole.

Can I be certain of these ideas? Absolutely not! To pretend otherwise would be to offer yet another ideology for others to follow. All I know for certain, is that whenever I sit quietly, take a breath and go 'inside', I suspend my immediate ambitions and defenses to experience what lies beneath, the sense of who I am changes dramatically. When I look back from this place to examine my recent thoughts, actions and intentions, I often find myself profoundly dejected by what I see. This isn't about guilt - a belief that I have failed to live up to some external expectation; it's a pervasive sense of shame that comes from knowing that I have been a traitor to my Self. My first impulse is to admonish myself and promise myself to 'do better'. But that's ridiculous – the replaying of an old program that my brain concocted to ward off the guilt implanted by others. The only sensible response I can make is to *be* my Self and for me, this continues to be a slow and incremental process. When I move back into the external world, the old fears still return and the well-rehearsed programs are always waiting to jump into the breach. That's just the way it is. I have never claimed to be complete, whole or enlightened. The important thing is that I am moving in a direction that urges me to examine what I have learned, dismantle my self-limiting programs and bring my Self more fully into the relational world.

Only when we recognize ourselves as conscious and purposeful beings can we begin to re-create the world in a way that supports our lives on this planet and affirms our inherent related-ness to the whole.

All in the Family

"Nothing can be changed until it's seen for what it is." This statement usually attributed to Fritz Perls, the father of Gestalt Therapy, implies there is actually something to be seen and the observer can, in fact, see. In other words, conscious and purposeful change begins with awareness. At an individual level, we must be aware; not only of our current circumstances, but also of how they came to be. This is the task of searching through the complexity of our own lives to discover the simple truths of our existence. If we cannot see the patterns of our past, the chances are we will go on repeating them, only to end up back in the same place. For the most part, these patterns did not originate within our own lives, but were handed down by parents who in turn, inherited them from their parents, and so on. In some cases these cross-generational influences are subtle and ambiguous; in others, they are so pronounced they are often attributed to genetic programming and by implication, beyond our control. Whatever form they take, they represent an intricate web of human relationships, past and present, which shape our lives from conception onwards. On the positive side, these legacies give distinction to our families and provide the rich fabric of our cultures. However, if left unseen, they are prescriptions that lock us into blindly repeating the legacies of the past, hanging on to the old beliefs while playing out our roles in an unconscious relational saga. As the good Doctor Fritz supposedly said – nothing can be changed until it's seen for what it is!

> *If we cannot see the patterns of our past, the chances are we will go on repeating them, only to end up back in the same place.*

Our primary concern here is not about facts, events or even individuals. The legacies of the past are created and handed down through relationships, and it is through our current relationships that we perpetuate the old motives, meanings and mythologies. To see ourselves in this relational matrix is to create the opportunity to make different choices. By revisiting and reflecting upon the circumstances of our own childhood, we can come to understand the degree to which our lives have been influenced by our earliest relational experiences, and how we continue to work from agendas that are not of our making. As a bonus, this illuminating exercise also makes it possible for us to better understand the lives of our children, from a place of curiosity, sensitivity and empathy.

When it comes to re-examining our personal learning histories, I believe the only qualified investigator is the authentic Self. To engage and retain the services of the Self in this project is remarkably simple, though rarely easy. In my own case, I learned how to hide and mask my authentic feelings from a very early age. Much later in life, like many other seekers of my generation, I set out on my 'search for Self" by participating in encounter groups, personal growth programs and various forms of psychotherapy. While I don't wish to discount such dedication to the cause, I've come to realize that direct access to the Self is actually a very natural process and available to all. In its most basic form, it's as simple as taking a breath and staying in touch with whatever happens. The breath opens up the energetic channel for the Self to find expression and, given this opportunity, the Self will respond accordingly. While it takes discipline and practice to set this process in motion, the inside voice gradually gains confidence and clarity to become the central intelligent guide. There are many well-established 'techniques' for bringing this about, but rather than divert from my theme at this point, I have chosen to include descriptions of these methods in the appendices of this book.

If you are still wondering what all this has to do with the day-to-day adventures of being with children, I can only ask for your continued indulgence. We are dealing here with the deep and hidden structures of human relationships, and I firmly believe that, unless we have some awareness of what is taking place at this level, we will be unable to offer young people what they now need. We cannot turn our attention to nurturing the development of another Self unless we are familiar with the development of our own, and can recognize the separation between them. Personally, I have found this to be a formidable and fascinating project that opens up unlimited opportunities and solutions, infinitely more effective than even the most elegant prescriptions designed by the most knowledgeable experts. If you're still anxious to know how this translates into parenting and teaching practices, please be assured this becomes the focus in the latter part of this book. Meanwhile, I will attempt to outline ways through which the Self may begin to explore its own developmental history.

We cannot turn our attention to nurturing the development of another Self unless we are familiar with the development of our own, and can recognize the separation between them.

There are many possible directions to take, but the most accessible point of departure is probably the winding trail that takes us back through the topography of our own family, from the present generation to those that went before. I'm not talking about mapping out a lifeless genealogy, although this certainly provides a useful framework. In its purest form, the Self exists in the moment, being concerned only with the lived-in experience. It is the 'true witness' and, given the freedom to access our senses and intellect, it becomes an astute and finely tuned

*With this awareness,
we have the choice of
either breaking free
from the old legacies
or passing whatever
we were given on to
our own children.
Without awareness,
we remain locked into
the second option.*

participant-observer. Its concern is not with the 'facts' as such, but with the subjective experiences of those involved in the action. The primary interests of the Self are relational, and from this perspective the history of a family becomes a history of lived-in relationships. When we examine these relationships, and what was passed down from one generation to the next, we begin to understand the context of our lives, how we have come to see ourselves as we do, and how we learned to be in relationships with others. With this awareness, we have the choice of either breaking free from the old legacies or passing whatever we were given on to our own children. Without awareness, we remain locked into the second option.

Jack Lee Rosenberg, the creator of Integrated Body Psychotherapy (IBP), refers to this learning heritage as the "Primary Scenario," and believes that conscious and self-directed change cannot occur unless we have a clear understanding of the relational context into which we were born. To this end, he has developed a powerful and highly effective procedure through which his clients are able to explore their personal histories across three generations, while remaining centered in their own experience of Self. From an IBP perspective, the authentic Self is experienced directly as a felt sense of well being in the body and the exploratory process is both cognitive and somatic. The reasons for bringing the body into the picture will, hopefully, become more apparent as we move on. Meanwhile, having used this method to review my own, and many other lives, I can readily attest to its effectiveness. To provide a framework, and illustrate the significance of early learning within our family of origin, I would like to pave the way by referring back to my own relational history.

If you would like more information on this topic and the work of Jack Rosenberg, I would urge you to read his book *Body, Self & Soul: Sustaining Integration*, published in 1985. Written in conjunction with Marjorie Rand and Diane Asay, this very readable text describes what I believe to be the most comprehensive and elegant system of psychotherapy available today.

The Scene is Set

I was born in the north of England at the beginning of the Second World War. Most historians would agree this event was a phenomenon of the twentieth century, but my thesis would suggest it was actually the outcome of countless choices made and actions taken, from the time we humans first became capable of consciously creating and selecting options on our own behalf. As it happened, I was born into a dichotomized world of 'bad guys' and 'good guys'. It was a time when the idea of being English was prominent in the minds of my caretakers, and traditional British values were considered to be the key to our national integrity and survival – Mr. Churchill told us so. Could there be any doubt that these beliefs and values would become firmly entrenched in my young psyche?

Prior to my conception, my working-class parents had dreamed of creating the perfect family unit – one boy, one girl and a semi-detached house in the suburbs. Their shared ambition was to raise the status of the family from its working class base to the more comfortable existence of a middle class lifestyle. When I was conceived, they were well on their way to attaining this objective. They had a five-year-old son and the money they needed for the down payment on a modest home in a lower middle-class part of town. My conception was carefully planned and my arrival eagerly anticipated. Then came the war.

My father was immediately drafted into the Air Force and my brother was 'evacuated' to live with an adoptive family in a rural community as a protection from the nightly raids of the German Luftwaffe. My paternal grandmother, who lived with the family, had already decided to move out rather than face the prospect of having yet another child in her life – she had struggled to raise eight of her own. My mother found herself alone, grieving the absence of her son, fearing for her husband's life and increasingly anxious about the prospect of raising two children without his support. Meanwhile, "Geraldine" lay quietly in the womb as the celebration of 'her' presence turned into doubt and anxiety. These conditions persisted throughout the second trimester of the pregnancy until two months before my 'due date,' circumstances changed once again. Quite by chance, my father was posted to a nearby air base and with his return to family life, both parents re-embraced the pregnancy and revived the old dream. So, from being wanted, I became unwanted and then, prior to my birth, I was wanted again.

Believe it or not, this 'wanted-unwanted' theme has continued to manifest itself throughout my relational life. The pattern is one in which I either engage in short-term superficial liaisons, or give myself away to those I most care about in a desperate attempt to keep them around. If others get too close, however, my automatic responses are to either back off or test the strength of their commitment by making unreasonable demands. Then, should they choose to distance themselves from me, I seduce them into coming back with well-tried and tested pleasing maneuvers – and so the dance goes on. While this tedious *pas de deux* might have served some purpose in warding off my early fears of rejection and abandonment, it has persistently sabotaged my attempts to bring my Self fully to the party. This defensive script became so entrenched in my life that I, along with many others, came to see it as feature of my personality, a reflection of my authentic Self. The most frustrating part is that, while I can now recognize it for what it really is and step in before too much damage is done, the original fears are still there and the old program is always primed and ready for action. Even in my most intimate relationship of forty-two years, this same disruptive routine can still kick in when things begin to go awry.

My World Before Birth

Developmentally, I may attribute my irrational fears and aberrant behaviors to some interruption in the early bonding between my mother and myself. Given what I've already written, this makes a lot of sense, but two questions need to be addressed. Is it possible I could have known about my mother's attitudinal and emotional shifts from my place in the womb? If this is so, why have I not been able use my adult insight to eradicate the problem?

The answer to the first question is undoubtedly "yes". The idea that children are aware through their pre-birth experiences, and can subsequently recall episodes of life in the womb, is neither new nor radical. In the early twentieth century, the eminent psychoanalyst Otto Rank spoke so convincingly on this subject in his book, *The Trauma of Birth*, that his even more famous colleague Sigmund Freud was moved to observe that this work represented the most important progress since the discovery of psychoanalysis. During the 1940s and 1950s, many other clinicians documented countless cases of pre-birth memory, most notably the British pediatrician Donald Winnicott. The first serious attempt to piece together an experiential account of life in the womb was made by Scottish psychiatrist R.D. Laing in his book, *The Facts of Life* published in 1976. For the most part, these early pioneers had neither the methodology nor the technology to support their speculations with verifiable data, but their clinical studies still make compelling reading.

In 1981, Thomas Verny established a landmark in the exciting new field of Pre-and Perinatal Psychology with the publication of his book, *The Secret Life of the Unborn Child*. Drawing upon a growing body of research, Verny cast aside the 'convenient' medical view of the fetus as a senseless biological object to present a fascinating picture of the unborn child as a sensitive and responsive being, engaged in an active relationship with the mother. His "Gestational Model" divides intrauterine life into six broad developmental phases. During the early stages of pregnancy, the information exchanged between mother and child is essentially physiological; being based upon biological shifts and generalized sensations. By the twenty-eighth week, however, the unborn child possesses the same functional neural circuits as the newborn infant. This makes it possible for the child to receive and differentiate among the many subtle messages received from the mother. This information is transmitted though an intricate network of neuro-hormonal pathways, linking the two beings in an intimate and synchronistic relationship. Experiences that were only sensations in the first trimester are systematically transformed into subtly differentiated emotional states and organized into specific patterns of response. Throughout the third trimester, the child becomes increasingly capable of receiving, differentiating, retaining and responding to complex information from many diverse sources, including a mother's thoughts and significant external events. The startling implications are that, rather than being a passive learner, the unborn child becomes a conscious and aware being, actively involved in creating his or her physical, emotional, intellectual and relational life.

When I first read Verny's book I was moved to tears. At the time, I could think of no rational reason for such an emotional response to a scholarly treatise, but the feelings were real, and oddly familiar. On reflection, I recognized them as being similar to the feelings I have when some hidden or disguised aspect of my Self rises to the surface to be acknowledged by another Self – a validation of something already known. Later, when I listed Verny's book as required reading for two of my university courses, it created a wave of excitement and speculation among students wearied by having to learn the classical theories of developmental psychology. As one hitherto reluctant male learner remarked, "My God! This stuff changes everything." Another student, a young mother, wanted to know why women needed a male scientist to tell them the truth of their own bodies?

Verny's picture of intrauterine life has been well supported by subsequent research, and I will touch on some of these findings a little later. Meanwhile, I believe my first question has been answered in the affirmative – the evidence suggests that I was indeed able to pick up on my mother's prenatal ambivalence from my place in the womb. To make matters even more simple, the accommodating Dr. Verny then goes on to address the second question regarding my inability to eradicate the sources of my self-defeating relational patterns – my 'pathology,' if you like.

In much of the early clinical work, psychotherapists noted how their patients' prenatal recollections related to experiences and events that occurred well before the emergence of the cognitive networks generally considered as the essential precursors of memory. In the light of such findings, Verny surmised that memory appears to be comprised of two functionally separate, though interrelated, systems. One is cerebral, or neurological memory and is made possible through the development of the central nervous system toward the end of the second trimester of pregnancy. The other, more basic, system is in place from conception onwards and operates at a biological, or cellular, level. This notion of "cellular memory" is based upon the 'holographic' principle that every cell knows what every other cell knows but also contributes additional information specific to that cell. Thirty years later, this proposition was supported through the work of Bruce Lipton, but at the time, it found little acceptance or interest in the scientific community.

The implications are that the critical elements of prenatal learning are not processed and stored within the cerebral networks of the brain but in the somatic structures of the body. Since such experiences are not created or mediated by the mind's cognitive operations, memories of these events can only be accessed through the body. Whatever interpretations the mind might attach to these experiences, their inherent integrity remains solid and untouched. This of course, would account for my failed attempts to eradicate my automatic relational responses by simply thinking about them; pathology explained, but not 'cured.'

On the more positive side, I no longer consider myself locked into this primitive pattern. Now I believe I have choices. Through therapeutic bodywork, I have learned that by inviting my body to explore and communicate its knowledge energetically, I can come to know a deeper level of Self, not as an idea floating around in my head, but as a felt sense of continuity and well-being in my body – just as Rosenberg suggested. This includes some understanding of the interruptions that occurred during those first two months in-utero, but it also informs me of something much more profound. Whoever I was before thoughts and words came along to complicate matters still lives in that same place, waiting to be seen and heard. This I believe is the essence of who I am, the non-negotiable being, the 'I' within the 'Me'. This is the voice that speaks from inner experience and urges me to act on my own behalf, and my separation from this voice creates the void that John Fowles refers to as the Nemo. The cellular memory of early interruptions or traumas will never be completely erased, but

Whoever I was before thoughts and words came along to complicate matters still lives in that same place, waiting to be seen and heard.

once identified and understood for what they are, the automatic defensive patterns can be arrested and modified through self-conscious action. To return to one of my earlier questions, I am suggesting that that the core human Self has always been there; the contribution of evolution has been to provide us with neurological equipment through which the voice of the Self can be heard, understood, and expressed in action. This I believe, is the source of our freedom.

Conversely, I also know something about the dangers of ignoring what the body has to say. I grew up believing I was the fun-seeking, well-meaning, though basically incompetent, person my mind had created – with a little help from family and friends. In my final undergraduate year, I was told how I could reshape this mental image by changing my thoughts and behaviors, so I did. Next to psychotropic medication, this technique has become the cornerstone of psychiatric practice across North America. It's now called "cognitive-behavior modification." Within a year I went from being a mediocre student among the beer-swilling ne'er-do-wells to become an aspiring academic with faculty connections and access to the Graduate Student Lounge. My self-esteem improved significantly – I still have the pre-and-post tests to prove it. I was a competitor, and basked in whatever recognition I could elicit from the academic elite. I even sent morsels of my achievements home for my parents to chew on. I had taken my first sniff of 'success' and I wanted more. For once in my meandering life, the pathway ahead was clear and the rewards were definitive and attainable.

With little concern for whatever was taking place on the inside, I pursued my dream, oblivious to the wordless voice and unaware of the price I was paying for my hearing deficit. When my body began to withdraw its support for my ambitions, I sought medical attention for the symptoms, but the underlying 'pathology' always returned in one form or another. Determined not to let my physical health stand in the way of progress, I made many attempts to change my lifestyle. I tried regular exercise, balanced diets and became an avid reader of popular health magazines but for some reason, the benefits always proved to be unsustainable. Only when I began regular sessions with a body-focused psychotherapist did I come to realize how hard I had been working to deny and repress what I most needed to know. In a nutshell, my body was a tightly held system of blocked and spluttering energy, the casualty of a life-long battle with a restless and fearful mind. "Get out of your head and come to your senses," my therapist would say, but I had to think a lot about that one. Putting my mind at ease and allowing my body to share its 'truth' is still a challenge but I now know that, with each incremental release, my body knows how to speak and my mind can be trained to listen. Piece by piece, the past trickles into the present as the memories, cerebral and somatic, blend into that which is me. I cannot change the past but, once my history is known and understood, I am free to change my response to it.

While support for Verny's Gestational Model has been steadily growing for the past three decades, there is one provocative question that remains to be explored. If cellular memory gives me access to my pre-cognitive history, and this information can seep into my conscious experience, how far back can I go? Verny's assertion that memories are encoded and stored within a single cell suggests that each ovum and sperm may carry specific messages from one generation to the next. I find it fascinating to consider how the egg destined to bring me into this world was actually in my mother's body when she was in her own mother's womb. Does this mean that aspects of Granny's life and history were stored in my egg as it waited to receive new messages from my mother, as well as those contained within the sperm so generously supplied by my father? I could speculate about this at length, but for present purposes, suffice it to say that logic and experience leaves me open to consider such a hypothesis.

Thirty years ago, the idea that 'lived-in' family experiences are passed down from one generation to the next through what Verny referred to as "organismic memory" would have been speculative, to say the least. To some extent, it still is. If we accept what scientists are now telling us, that human consciousness is a definitive element within the universe, all we are really talking about is basic genetics with a neuro-hormonal twist. Could this be the key to our understanding of such diverse unexplained phenomena as intuition, past-life recall, near-death experiences, ESP and Carl Jung's notion of the collective unconscious? Maybe so, but more specific to the present discussion, we have here a scientific foundation for believing that conscious material is an integral part of the genetic package passed along

The implications are that every child comes into this world carrying a distilled version of all the learning and experience that has gone before... Perhaps the Dalai Lama's assertion that all children know more than their parents is not simply Buddhist rhetoric.

from one generation to the next. With reference to my comments at the beginning of this chapter, the implications are that every child comes into this world carrying a distilled version of all the learning and experience that has gone before. Perhaps the Dalai Lama's assertion that all children know more than their parents is not simply Buddhist rhetoric.

To return to my 'unwanted' developmental theme, research findings over the past thirty years have become increasingly consistent and unequivocal – kids who are not wanted at conception and through pregnancy display a wide range of emotional, intellectual, behavioral and relational difficulties. With twenty-five percent of all births being aborted world wide, and the increase in the number of babies born to uncommitted adults in western nations, we can only wonder about the numbers of children who enter this world with a deep sense of being unwanted, unwelcome and unacceptable. My own experience, including the research I conducted in designing a children's mental health system for the Province of Alberta, certainly confirms that 'unwanted' children are significantly over represented in North American juvenile justice and mental health systems. At the broader level, psychoanalyst John Sonne, Professor of Psychiatry at Robert Wood Johnson School of Medicine, is convinced that this trend is a significant contributor to the dehumanization and social regression in western cultures. My point is, we all receive messages in-utero and this information is carefully locked away in our cerebral and somatic memory banks for future reference. In my case, the "unwanted" message was relatively weak and distinctly

Kids who are not wanted at conception and through pregnancy display a wide range of emotional, intellectual, behavioral and relational difficulties.

transitory, yet undeniable.

My partner's in-utero experience was a little more sinister, however. When her pending arrival was confirmed, her father urged his wife to abort the pregnancy. After some initial hesitation, she resisted his appeals, but throughout the first trimester, the life of her would be daughter hung in the balance. Without going into details, Judith who is a practicing psychotherapist, remains convinced that this early message accounts for her pervasive sense of insecurity and her life long questions about her legitimacy in the world. The available clinical evidence clearly supports her beliefs.

The Controversial Issue of Abortion

Abortion is of course, the ultimate statement of rejection and abandonment. It is also a hotly contested religious, moral, social and political issue. This should not stop us from examining how the unborn child might respond to such messages, from initial parental ambivalence to failed attempts to terminate the pregnancy. Psychologist David Chamberlain, arguably the most prolific contributor to the field of pre- and perinatal psychology in recent years, has written extensively on this and many other related topics. A selective overview of his work can be found in a special issue of the *Journal of Prenatal and Perinatal Psychology and Health*. I consider this volume to be a classic, and as an educator believe it should be required reading for any student of developmental psychology.

In his review of cases of attempted but failed abortions, Chamberlain cites numerous studies to show how repressed memories of such events can have serious life long consequences. Included in this review, he tells the story of Australian psychiatrist Graham Farrant, who through his own search for Self, discovered how his mother had attempted to abort him with a combination of medication and hot baths. When he asked his 79-year old mother about this, she denied it completely before bursting into tears. Later she claimed he couldn't possibly know this because she had never told a living soul about her 'secret'. Chamberlain also documents the findings of Canadian psychologist Andrew Feldmar, who treated four youths, each of whom attempted suicide on numerous occasions at the same time each year. These gestures occurred on, or close to, the anniversary dates when their mothers attempted to abort them. None of these young men had any conscious knowledge of the attempted abortions until it was revealed through the course of therapy.

Even more disturbing is the study conducted by John C. Sonne. In his examination of the two youths responsible for the 1999 massacre at Columbine High School in the United States, he noted that the 'clinical profiles' of both boys were typical of abortion survivors. The common features of such profiles include: perceiving oneself as an outcast; a sense of being incurable – genetically flawed; a deeply rooted lack of trust in others; insatiable attention seeking; intense anger directed inward and outward; and suicide ideation and gestures. One of the youngsters in this study actually made a video recording prior to the killings that contained the Shakespearean quotation – "Good wombs have borne bad sons." (p.19). According to Sonne's interpretation of the video message, the young killer was saying, "My mother damaged me when I was in her womb, and I have murderous feelings toward her." (p.19). Rather than killing his mother however, he went out and killed others before turning his rage upon himself and committing suicide. Based upon this examination and other related studies, Sonne predicts that the prevalence of violent and murderous acts by young people will continue to escalate in a culture where "the multigenerational transmission of the threat of being aborted" is prevalent. (p.20). In a later article, he goes on to suggest that the primal fear of annihilation that exists in all of us has become a major contributor to psychological and social unrest around the globe. I wonder how the policy makers, planners and social engineers would respond if they ever stopped to consider such a proposition?

I am also aware of the many documented cases of 'spontaneous abortion' in which the fetus is considered to have terminated gestation by withdrawing the biochemical support necessary to sustain the pregnancy. We can only speculate about why and how such decisions might be made in-utero, but we can be sure that they would not be made upon moral, religious or political grounds. Where mother makes the call, my only concern is that the decision to abort should be made in awareness, and that includes understanding what is taking place in her womb.

With this in mind, there are a number of programs across North America designed to encourage and support mothers in communicating their decision to the unborn child, allowing their thoughts and feelings to be known and expressed. Given support and understanding, most women find their own way to say what needs to be said – some write poems, some paint pictures, some meditate, and some create interactive dialogues. Regardless of the particular method, such communication allows the mother to deal directly with what might otherwise be repressed and left unresolved. We can only speculate about how this information might be received on the inside, but I firmly believe that open and honest communication between one human being and another, particularly in matters of life and death, is intrinsically beneficial to both parties. At least, we can be assured that an infant in the first trimester of a pregnancy has not collected the psychological baggage that keeps most adults in fear and denial of their mortality. In this regard, you may find the following story of interest.

Some years ago, while attending a Pre and Perinatal Conference, I came upon a small huddle of dedicated listeners as a middle-aged woman, a psychologist by trade, told the remarkable story of her own abortion experience. At the age of nineteen, in her second year of university, she was shocked to discover she was pregnant. Four months earlier, she had been diagnosed as having Multiple Sclerosis and assumed that the early signs of pregnancy were symptoms of this debilitating disease. Along with the father, her husband-to-be, she sat for many hours considering the prospects of parenthood, and together they decided to terminate the pregnancy and keep this decision as a secret between themselves. They married three years later while still in graduate school, and given there were no indications to support the M.S. diagnosis, they planned to have at least one child before she began her professional career. Their son, Michael, was born ten months later. On his eleventh birthday, they were sitting at home after supper looking through an album of photographs taken at various times throughout the boy's life. The parents were surprised by his ability to recall details of the events depicted, and as psychologists, they were fascinated by his personal accounts. Being a specialist in early child development, his mother showed him a picture taken shortly after birth and asked if he could recall anything about that time in his life. When he told them he had only "hazy" memories, they accepted this without further questions, but his next comment was as unpredictable as it was startling. While continuing to gaze, seemingly absent mindedly, at his first baby picture, he said, "I was here before, you know. It just wasn't the right time."

The Prenatal Learner

Moving beyond the anecdotal, empirical research has given us much to think about over the past twenty years, challenging our old beliefs and offering fresh perspectives on life before birth. New technologies have made it possible for us to actually witness the moment of union between sperm and ovum, and observe the fetus throughout its intrauterine development. Thanks to the dedication of pioneers like Verny and Chamberlain, we have come to see the unborn child as a sentient relational being constantly moving toward higher levels of consciousness. We now know that babies dream while still in the womb, indicating the emergence of subconscious activity. We know that newborns can recognize words and music presented prior to birth, including the distinctive sounds of parental voices and passages read from Dr. Seuss. On this note, you might be interested to know that unborn babies like classical music, dislike hard rock and display a definite preference for Mozart over Beethoven. We also know that language patterns are learned from the mother in utero, not as syntax and grammatical sequences, but as characteristic rhythms and cadences recognized prior to birth and imitated afterwards.

The data generated through these and many other studies, reveal that our earliest learning is 'holistic' rather than incremental. In other words, the information is grasped in the form of complete sensory experiences, rather than discrete pieces taken in sequentially and classified cerebrally. This implies that the organism as a whole is engaged in the learning process, receiving information through all sensory apparatus, sending out responses, and monitoring the effects of those responses on the environment. This multimodal experiential learning style becomes clearly evident after birth through the infant's ability to recognize complex external stimuli such as human faces and the distinctive sound patterns of a human voice.

This being the case, I am left wondering why educators continue to separate the knowledge from the knower by focusing almost exclusively on the incremental and sequential learning style of the neo-cortex. I assume they are obsessed with filling the brain with abstractions of the external world because that's how we define 'education' and that's how they became qualified to 'teach'. From my own experience in schools, it's abundantly clear that the child's inherent capacity to learn 'holistically' is not only ignored, it is systematically eradicated in the service of intellectual-cognitive development and, of course, classroom management. If you are interested in how this tragedy unfolds, you may wish to take a look at George Leonard's insightful work, *Education and Ecstasy*

To take this issue even further, Joseph Chiltern Pearce, in his book *Evolution's End*, argues that our failure to integrate the learning of our primary universal experiences with the intellectual capacities of the neo-cortex has brought the evolution of our species to a shuddering halt. In this fascinating analysis, he identifies the heart as the central organ of learning for the senses and emotions – an idea that is gaining increasing recognition through the advent of computer imaging technology. While Pearce penetrates much deeper into the matter, my modest suggestion is that, by blending these two distinctive learning styles, we open up communication between the intuitive and cognitive, thereby creating an opportunity to explore the fullness of our human potential. Alternatively, if we continue to cram the intellectual system with more external information, we will only ensure that our intellect and intelligence, our minds and our bodies, will remain steadfastly apart. David Chamberlain's assertion that "the womb is a school, and all children attend" (p.190.b) takes us to the core of the issue. In contrast to our formal educational factories, the "classwomb" is, by design, a supportive, nurturing environment that responds to the unborn child as a full-time student in the University of Being.

Above all, the research of the past twenty or so years has confirmed that the essential nature of intrauterine life is indeed relational. From the beginning, whatever mother experiences, her baby also experiences. When she is happy and at one with the world, her baby basks in the same emotion. When she rests, the contented baby settles down with her, and when she dances, her invisible partner joins in the fun. On the other side, if she feels anxious or stressed, the baby experiences the same anxiety. If she feels unloved, unsupported and un-cared for, the child sinks into her desolation. And if she resents or denies the pregnancy, her baby will feel unsure about the "rightness" of his or her own existence. All of this is made possible through the placenta. What was once considered to be a simple protective device for the child's safety and comfort is now understood to be an active organ that transfers information back and forth within a complex interdependent biological, emotional, psychological and 'spiritual' union.

From the beginning, whatever mother experiences, her baby also experiences. When she is happy and at one with the world, her baby basks in the same emotion.

At the biological level, the connection between maternal health and fetal health is obvious and the benefits of good nutrition, healthy exercise and regular medical check-ups are well known and widely accepted. By the same token, if mother takes drugs, the baby takes the same drugs. Alcohol consumed at the time of conception can result in craniofacial abnormalities, and continued drinking increases the likelihood of Fetal Alcohol Syndrome. If mother lights up a cigarette, the baby smokes with her. In this regard, researcher Michael Lieberman has shown how unborn children will often become agitated when mother even thinks about having a cigarette. Subsequent research has demonstrated that prenatal exposure to cigarette smoking significantly lowers scores on pre-school tests of cognition and receptive language skills. Although the data are often scant and untrustworthy, we can confidently expect similar, or more serious, consequences from ingesting any of a wide range of prescription and 'recreational' drugs. In North America we live in a drug-dependent society, and even those substances considered to be relatively safe for the mother, may well turn out to be embryo-toxic with tragic consequences. Add to this our use of genetically modified foods along with the household and environmental teratogens that pollute our modern world and we begin to realize the extent of the problem. The trouble is, we can only see the tip of the iceberg. While the speculations and predictions are profoundly disturbing, the long-term effects on the physical, emotional, psychological and relational development of children remain largely unknown and unexplored. Given what we do know, it's alarming to note that over eighty percent of pregnant and lactating women in North America are given drugs as part of their routine medical care. Of course, the pharmaceutical industry is delighted with this arrangement, and since the drug companies now fund most research, it will likely stay this way until some catastrophe, like the Thalidomide debacle of the 1960's, brings us back to our senses. In my view however, none of this will really change until we come to realize that our place in nature is as purposeful participants, and our pitiful attempts to manipulate the universal order for our immediate gratification will always come back to haunt us.

Our Life in the Womb

Within the continuum of nature's design, the womb is where we first learn how to be in relationship with another human being. If nature is allowed to prevail, we come to know how it feels to be acknowledged, cared for and loved without conditions. Step by step, we learn how to express our own needs and wants, while responding to our partner's constantly shifting moods, activities and experiences. Our most predominant concern is that mother be 'there', fully present and engaged in what is taking place between us. The presence of mother's Self is the invitation we need to bring our own emerging Selves to the contact boundary. We learn how to tolerate her occasional absences, secure in the knowledge that she will be there when needed. Extended absence on the other hand, triggers our most primal fear of abandonment – a threat to our survival. The assurances we seek are essentially energetic, a simple wordless knowing that mother is around and that we are inextricably connected. All children love attention, and as our awareness develops we enjoy being spoken to directly. When this happens we connect with our hearts, our cardiac rhythms responding not to the words themselves, but to the energetic qualities of the message. We open our hearts to mother's voice, listening and responding well before we have the ears to hear. What we experience are the subtle vibrations of sound upon our skin, our most sensitive and receptive organ. In the words of David Chamberlain, we live "in the sound waves of (our) mother's body and in the tidal flow of her emotions, sparked by thoughts and experiences." (190 b). All of this is as nature intends, laying the foundations for our future physical, emotional and relational development. Here in the womb, we experience the interconnectedness, the honesty and the intimacy that we will spend much of our lives seeking to find in the outside world. If all goes according to plan, we will begin that quest with the confidence and the resources necessary to make it happen.

> *Here in the womb, we experience the interconnectedness, the honesty and the intimacy that we will spend much of our lives seeking to find in the outside world.*

The flow of nature is beset with interruptions, and so it is with every human life. Rather than being impediments in the developmental process, early interruptions are essential if the fledgling Self is to build strength and resilience from the inside out. Those times in the womb when mother is not immediately available, her emotions are disturbing, and her thoughts less than loving are essential aspects of the learning process. Significant problems only arise when the interruptions are so prolonged or severe that an injured Self recoils and becomes dedicated to its own protection. At the biological level, consider Bruce Lipton's description of individual cells moving toward closure and systems shutting down.

Becoming Responsible

I have already identified aspects of the mother-child relationship that might interfere with the developmental process, but there are also external interruptions that can be particularly painful, even violent. While modern technology has allowed us to observe uterine life in startling detail, medical practices continue to invade this sacred place with arrogant insensitivity. For the most part, physicians still regard pregnancy as a medical state and consider the unborn infant to be less than human, incapable of experiencing discomfort and feeling pain. Yet the evidence suggests the very opposite. Sonogram images have clearly shown babies recoiling and becoming motionless when needles are inserted into the womb for amniocentesis. In some cases, they have been observed reaching out to grasp the needle itself, even though their eyes are firmly closed. If this visible evidence can be casually dismissed, the medical world is still a long way from recognizing and responding to the complex mental, emotional and relational aspects of life in the womb.

If you are curious about why medical practitioners have tended to ignore the findings of prenatal and perinatal research, I can offer two possible suggestions. In the first place such conclusions are glaringly inconvenient, requiring not only a change in the way medics go about their business, but demanding a fundamental shift in attitude. Secondly, most practitioners are completely unaware of such research. The medical journals have shown little interest in publishing this material, medical schools have chosen to look the other way, and medical research seems far more concerned with improving current technology or developing more drugs for the market place. If your curiosity urges you to ask why this is so, I will leave you to draw your own conclusions. Meanwhile, back to the classwomb...

If what we learn in the womb lays the foundation for our future relationships, then mother is indeed, the formative figure in our lives through childhood and beyond.

If what we learn in the womb lays the foundation for our future relationships, then mother is indeed, the formative figure in our lives through childhood and beyond. Whether we continue to build upon these early patterns or seek resolution and change through our subsequent relationships, mother's influence will never be deleted from our cellular core. "Tell me about your relationship with your mother," has become a cliché attributed to stereotypical psychoanalysts, but without this information all therapists are really working in the dark. In bodywork and the so-called 'regression' therapies the trail almost always leads back to encounters with the "Big M", sometimes loving sometimes resentful and sometimes openly hostile. For girls, the synergy of life in the womb prepares the way for womanhood. After birth the primary bond is put to the test as the daughter moves from relating to mother as an object to recognizing her as a separate human being, another woman. On the other side I know men's primary issues are meant to revolve around the figure of the father, however, the hero's return journey also takes him straight back to mother, whether in tears tantrums or terror. How can it be any other way?

Given this, I am sometimes accused by my students of "mother bashing". They demand to know why fathers are always let off the hook. Their interpretation is: - If mother is assumed to be responsible for what takes place in utero, can she also be blamed for whatever happens later? This usually sets up an emotionally charged debate with the battle lines drawn roughly, though not exclusively between the sexes. When the willingness to listen has been restored to acceptable educational levels I use my tenuous authority to redirect the remaining energy into a discussion on the differences between the concepts of 'responsibility' and 'blame'. This in turn, paves the way for me to review the presented material and clarify my own position. For me it's not about "mother bashing." My own mother, bless her heart, deserves better than that.

At the broadest level I am suggesting that through the union of sperm and ovum, we are conceived into a pre-existing web of relationships. Once established in the womb however, mother becomes the nexus from which our own relational matrix will gradually emerge. From this place, she acts as the medium, or interpreter, passing on to us her own relational history. What we absorb are not the relationships themselves, but mother's responses to her own connections close and distant, past and present. In this sense her level of responsibility – or response-ability – depends upon the degree to which she is able to see these influences and if necessary, free herself from any self-defeating patterns and entanglements. In other words, personal responsibility begins with awareness and is expressed through the ability and willingness to take self-directed action.

This does not mean mother is to 'blame' for her lack of awareness, or for her failure to provide her unborn child with the most optimal learning environment, whatever that might look like. To varying degrees, we are all lacking in awareness and constantly find ourselves in circumstances that limit our self-volition. Professionally I have come across many parenting tragedies, although I continue to believe that for the most part, parents do the very best they can, given their own learning histories and personal resources. Nevertheless, I usually take the position that parents should be held accountable for their actions, knowing full well that I am making an external judgment based upon an external expectation. According to my definition, response-ability, the ability to respond, is an internal matter being concerned with the conscious actions of an informed Self. It's more about intention and integrity than about incrimination.

Like some of my recalcitrant students you may choose to dismiss my definition. My only purpose is to briefly review my perspective and leave you to your own interpretations. Yet there is one question I have deliberately avoided. Regardless of circumstances, is awareness a matter of choice and lack of awareness a way of consciously or unconsciously avoiding self-responsible actions? I leave this for you to consider. Meanwhile, I will move on to address the second aspect of my students' concern – the significance of the father in the life of the unborn child.

Taking biology out of the equation, father (or mother's primary partner) has a critical part to play throughout the pregnancy. He or she usually provides the closest link in mother's relational network, and what takes place between the two adults profoundly affects what is taking place in the womb. This is the crucible from which mother draws her sense of well being; her feelings of being loved and cared for, and her view of herself as a mother. Unlike the distilled remnants of history, the emotions she experiences through her primary relationship are immediate powerful and available to the newcomer from one moment to the next. Forgive me if I say again, you can only give to an Other what you already have for your Self.

In the early stages mother's partner may appear to be one step removed from the center of the action, but child rearing is by design, a shared project and this is as true during pregnancy as it is through the adolescent years. According to this design, what happens between a mother and her unborn child confirms the continuity of connectedness through the transition from the spiritual into the physical. Her relationship with her partner is the context in which the infant learns about connections that are distinctively human. If this relationship is open and loving, a meeting of Selves, the newcomer will move into life with trust and confidence. To the degree this relationship is closed or hostile, the infant will either test the parental tolerance or withdraw into a place of protection. If mother has no significant relationship, the child's opportunity to learn is almost certainly compromised. My position is not moralistic or idealistic; I'm simply trying to establish the conditions in which children learn about human relationships.

If this relationship is open and loving, a meeting of Selves, the newcomer will move into life with trust and confidence… If mother has no significant relationship, the child's opportunity to learn is almost certainly compromised.

Apart from confirming the popular belief that happy Moms tend to have happy babies, research now shows how there can be a direct connection between the unborn child and at least one person on the 'outside' – a second relationship. Even in the first trimester the fetus will respond to such external stimulation as tapping or stroking mother's belly. As time goes on, these stimulus response encounters become increasingly interactive as the child senses a familiar presence on the outside. The more frequent the interaction, the more finely tuned this process becomes, and the kind of relationship the parties wish to have becomes increasingly known to both. While the communication methods may be rudimentary, the energetic connection contains a wealth of information including the outside person's thoughts and feelings about the child. Simply by communicating directly, he or she acknowledges the 'insider's' existence as a significant and separate being. The sound of the voice and the quality of the touch communicate feelings and intentions that may well lay the foundations for a relationship that will profoundly impact both of their lives. From a broader perspective, this also implies that, prior to birth, children are already learning about where they fit in the spectrum of immediate relationships beyond their union with mother – their place in the family.

In this sense, the unborn child is part of the parental relationship, and the interaction between the two adults is also experienced on the inside. As with mother, the partners' levels of awareness and involvement are key factors influencing the quality of life in the womb. With this in mind parents who are aware and self-responsible will share their thoughts and feelings openly, knowing the infant will not be deceived by empty words, contrived thoughts, or fictitious

The mind can distort whatever it wishes but the body knows only the 'truth' and communicating with an unborn child is a wonderful opportunity to explore what it means to be authentic.

feelings. The mind can distort whatever it wishes but the body knows only the 'truth' and communicating with an unborn child is a wonderful opportunity to explore what it means to be authentic. Learning to be honest at this stage is also good preparation and practice in the art of conscious parenting. Manipulating children with concocted 'truths' may seem justified at the time, but in the long run this serves only to undermine the integrity and trust between parent and child. At the prenatal stage, it's simply impossible.

The attitude of parents toward the pregnancy, including their hopes and wishes for the child, is particularly relevant. Left unacknowledged and unexplored they can remain as secret messages stuck in the unconscious, while covertly expressing themselves through attitudes and actions – a hidden agenda if you like. What the child experiences is confusion and doubt. Only by bringing them into the open can these messages be examined and, possibly, reconsidered. Similarly, hidden fears and concerns will continue to eat away from the inside until they are brought into consciousness. The object of this exercise is not that parents should abandon their hopes and dismiss any fears they judge to be undesirable; only that they become aware of these expectations or beliefs and recognize where they come from. Awareness is the foundation of personal responsibility and as a rule parents will quickly amend or relinquish any agenda that is clearly not in a child's best interests. Of course there are exceptions, but my experience in working with multigenerational family patterns clearly indicates that it's the unconscious, or secret stuff that does by far the most damage.

As parents we all have some agenda for our children but without conscious awareness, even the most laudable intentions can backfire. In their book, *I'll Never Do to My Kids What My Parents Did to Me*, Thomas and Eileen Paris describe in some detail what can happen when parents, or prospective parents, react against the way they themselves were parented. Unaware they are dealing with their own childhood injuries they strive to reverse the old parenting behaviors - to do things differently. The covert messages that were passed on to them, such as "good children don't get angry" or "failure is a sign of weakness," along with deeply entrenched feelings such as guilt, abandonment and unworthiness, continue to operate behind the scenes. Left unseen this pervasive legacy inevitably seeps through and parents find themselves unwittingly repeating the very strategies they so desperately wish to avoid. Despite their best intentions they can become emotionally controlling, overprotective, critical and judgmental, or overly permissive - just as their own parents were. And they can end up handing the same package over to the next generation.

In psychological language this is called "repetition compulsion". As a child I had great respect for my father, but as I grew older I became offended by some of his enduring traits and behaviors. His negativity about the weather, his tendency to exaggerate the symptoms of minor illnesses, and his lack of discretion around basic bodily functions were high on my list of complaints. Feedback however sensitively delivered, only served to reinforce the undesirable behaviors so I gave up and vowed never to take on these characteristics of my most significant male

Unaware they are dealing with their own childhood injuries they strive to reverse the old parenting behaviors - to do things differently... Despite their best intentions they can become emotionally controlling, overprotect-tive, critical and judg-mental, or overly perm-issive - just as their own parents were. And they can end up handing the same package over to the next generation.

model. Sparing you the details my failure can best be summarized by the question frequently posed by my long-suffering partner, "Why do I feel as if I'm living with your father?" Why, indeed? By the same token, our daughter used to wonder why she often felt guilty after buying clothes even when given full permission to make her own decisions. Now she understands that such license carried my unspoken expectation that she would make the 'right' choice – not too expensive, age appropriate and certainly not 'revealing'. At her age my clothes were always bought for me; they were never what I would have chosen, they were embarrassingly cheap and, among my peers, did nothing to reflect my burgeoning masculinity. My own kids would never have to endure such humiliation. Now over forty my daughter still feels the old twinge of guilt whenever she buys the clothes she really likes.

Whose Little Girl Was I?

Having drifted back into personal reflections, allow me to share with you some of the hidden agendas within my own family history. I've already had a lot to say about messages of being wanted or unwanted and, for the time being will let that discussion stand. I also revealed that I was expected to be a girl at birth, and this I would like to discuss in more detail.

Let me begin by saying that my parent's preference for a Geraldine over a Gerald was never openly stated and discussed, at least not with me, until I was well into my teens. It was my mother who really wanted a daughter, someone she could relate to as a female in a male dominated world. My father was fairly neutral on the issue, but agreed that a baby girl would be a nice balance for the family. I can't honestly say I was aware of this in the 'waiting-womb,' although I have found some amusement imagining myself becoming aware of my developing genitalia and thinking, "Oh God, what am I supposed to do with this little bundle?" What I can say is that I was treated like a girl for the first year or so of my life – my baby pictures remain as testimony to the deception. I was always dressed in pink, my head was a mass of delicate curls and I learned how to be 'cute' with strangers. "Oh what a beautiful baby girl," they would say, and my mother would beam back in appreciation. In my father's absence, my brother became the only guardian of my maleness. "He's not my sister, he's my baby brother," he would tell them with churlish schoolboy indignation. Eventually, even he gave up, leaving the infantile cross-dresser to perform alone.

I don't consider myself to have been severely injured through my participation in mother's secret fantasy and my sheer size, (I was over ten pounds at birth) ensured that the pretense would be fragile and short lived. On the other hand, my physical and behavioral male characteristics were slow to develop, and the family photo album depicts an infant becoming increasingly sullen, scowling at the camera and avoiding contact with others. In *The Continuum Concept*, Jean Leidloff talks about a child's inherent sense of 'rightness.' When the world gives out the message that something is 'wrong', that things are not as they should be, this inner sense is compromised and children will do whatever they can to make themselves right again. Within 'the continuum' they know that mother's love and attention is essential for their survival. The problem with being the wrong sex is that nothing can be done to change this fundamental flaw. Fortunately both parents loved me, and on the surface at least, they expressed both pride and pleasure in their two boys. If my mother continued to feel less than satisfied with my gender she certainly kept this to herself. I was also taken under the wing of my maternal grandmother who was determined to mould me into a 'man of distinction.'

Yet throughout my younger adult years, I was always reluctant to explore and express the fullness of my masculinity and found myself more at ease in the company of women. When men got into their macho stuff I viewed them with disdain, regarding them as testosterone driven zombies with their brains and sensitivities hovering somewhere between their navels and their knee caps. Oddly enough I was captain of my High School rugby team, recognized for my bull headed antics on the field and considered by my coaches to have professional potential. But on the inside I was always faking it, looking for token acceptance in a world I secretly disliked – or feared. Among my male peers, I was certainly a leader, and the old family album contains many pictures of me standing front and centre, surrounded by a gaggle of grinning supporters. My leadership was more about controlling the masculine imperative than exploring its potentials. The prospect of following some other brute into the forbidden depths of the adolescent male psyche was to be avoided at all costs.

As I suggested above, the 'wrong sex' message is a tough one to deal with since short of surgical intervention, there is nothing that will change this physical reality. In my professional practice I have worked with many people, young and old, who have struggled to come to terms with this legacy. While some rebelled by exaggerating and flaunting the stereotypical characteristics of their allotted sex, most did their best to please their parents by taking on the role of the more desired gender always knowing at some level they would ultimately fail the test. Apart from the confusion this brings into subsequent relationships, wrong sex children usually experience a deep sense of personal unworthiness and futility, stemming from a belief that they are not 'right' and there's not a thing they can do about it. In developing a negative view of their own gender they establish a negative view of themselves that can seep into many areas of their lives.

Wrong sex children usually experience a deep sense of personal unworthiness and futility, stemming from a belief that they are not 'right' and there's not a thing they can do about it.

Although I consider my own case to be relatively innocuous, my search through our family history did uncover one very interesting piece of information. Across three generations in my mother's family, there was a marked negative attitude toward men simmering beneath the surface of most significant relationships. This raises the possibility that my mother was unknowingly responding to a prejudice passed down from her parents and grandparents. Since she died some years ago, it's impossible for me to check this out but when I reflect on what I learned about men through the perceptions and judgments of my mother, it's not difficult to draw such a conclusion.

I also uncovered evidence indicating that my mother's unspoken desire for her children to rise above our working class status was not of her own making. The seeds of this ambition were sown two generations earlier when the family slipped down the social ladder and she became the unwitting inheritor of the recovery plan. Again I'm not implying it was wrong for my mother to want better things for her kids - quite the contrary. The problem was that she, my father, my brother and myself were all part of a design that was never placed on the kitchen table. Had we been aware of it we may still have gone along with the overall intent but I, for one would have done things very differently. On the other hand I would not have followed the advice offered by the English Poet Laureate Phillip Larkin who came from my own hometown and grew up in circumstances similar to my own. On the subject of parental legacies, he wrote:

They fuck you up, your Mum and Dad.
They may not mean to, but they do.
They fill you with the faults they had,
then add some extras, just for you.
But they were fucked up in their turn,
by fools in old time hats and coats,
who half the time were soppy, stern
and half at one another's throats.
Man hands on misery to man.
It deepens like a coastal shelf
Get out as quickly as you can
And don't have any kids yourself.

Tabling the Agenda

Even with the best will in the world, parental agendas may be difficult to uncover since they are often buried deep in the psyche of each individual. Once revealed they usually turn out to be expectations the child will provide something missing from the life of the parent, an unmet need or a frustrated ambition. Therein lays the heart of the tragedy. It is simply impossible for a child to satisfy such desires, leaving all concerned to experience only frustration and failure. In effect it turns out to be a complete reversal of nature's script in which the adult is supposed to address the developmental needs of the child.

However trite and self evident this might seem, my work over the years has led me to believe that this destructive dynamic lies at the core of most chronically troubled parent-child relationships. Professionals who attempt to intervene in such relationships without fully understanding how this mechanism works are more than likely to compound the problem. Even when parents do become aware of the underlying motivation they don't necessarily take personal ownership of the problem and move toward some form of resolution. Assisting parents to understand that the ball is now in their and supporting them in making decisions on their own behalf, are essential aspects of any effective counseling or therapy. With this in mind I would like to outline how my partner and I begin to address this matter in our professional practice.

In creating a comprehensive 'primary scenario' with each client we pursue three interrelated avenues of enquiry. The questions we use are derived from Rosenberg's model and this procedure is standard practice within the framework of Integrative Body Psychotherapy (IBP). The first, *Were you wanted?* leads us into an examination of all the possibilities and potentials outlined earlier in this chapter. At the deepest level we are interested in that person's sense of legitimacy in the world, of being valued by others as a worthy human being. The second, *Who wanted you?* identifies the location of the parental agenda. The third strikes the gong; *What were you wanted for?* With a little introspection and a felt sense in the body, some clients are able to identify the expectations, reflect on their childhood struggle to comply and recognizing the hopelessness of their task begin the work of unhooking themselves from the bondage. Others, those with the most work to do, don't even understand the question. The overall purpose in asking these questions is not to elicit simple answers and move on; it is an invitation to become aware of how our most primary relational influences continue to shape the nature of our lives. In our work, this is a major exploratory theme that extends throughout the course of therapy but these simple questions are highly relevant to anyone who seeks self-understanding. Ask them of yourself – you may be surprised, even enlightened, by your answers.

Spelled out in detail, there is an infinite number of possible responses to the critical question, ?' What were you wanted for? Over the years, I have listened to many intriguing plots and sagas. Once the specifics of character and circumstance are removed from the story however, these familial conspiracies tend to fall into particular categories; what Rosenberg refers to as 'hidden or secret themes'. The 'unwanted child' and the 'wrong gender child' are two of the most recurring examples but there are a number of others that emerge with significant frequency.

In our own work we often come across people whose job in their family was, and still is, to bring their parents together. This occurs in situations where one or both parents decide to become pregnant in the hope that a child will somehow resolve their on going relational difficulties. The sheer impossibility of this assignment is obvious, although the number of children and adults who continue to struggle might surprise you, desperately trying to bring harmony into a troubled parental relationship. While these children might end up in the helping professions their basic motivation is not really about others at all - it's about their own survival. From conception onwards children inherently know their lives are in the hands of their caretakers, and any threat to this arrangement is a matter of life or death. Defined by Rosenberg as the 'baby-as-glue' theme, this is just one of many possible patterns that lie within the secret lives of families. If you wish to examine these more fully, Rosenberg offers an interesting typology in his book *Body, Self & Soul: Sustaining Integration*.

The point I want to underscore is that, to some extent, we all had a job to do within our family of origin. In some cases the expectations were clearly stated with reasons disclosed and understood by all. The problems arise when a child struggles to meet hopelessly impossible expectations within an agenda that remains unknown and unacknowledged. These subtle programs may be embedded in cross generational patterns, existing relational networks or unsatisfied parental needs and aspirations, but they all have the same life debilitating effect. The major problem is not the agenda itself but the secrecy that surrounds it, particularly where that secret is protected by a parent's conscious belief that he or she is acting in the child's best interests. It may be perfectly fine for a father to dream about his unborn son playing in the National Hockey League, but if it becomes the boy's job to fulfill his father's unrealized athletic ambitions, both Selves are compromised. Most obviously, the lad is denied the opportunity to create his own career pathway, but the impact upon the Self goes much deeper. By the same token, there's nothing inherently wrong with a mother finding comfort in having her baby in her arms – quite the opposite. But if the infant is expected to provide her with the love she never received from her own parents or through the relationship with her partner, the same destructive die is cast. In both cases the incomplete Self of the parent consumes the fledgling Self of the child.

The most common developmental problem found in children born into powerful parental agendas is that they fail to acquire a sense of being able to act purposefully on their own behalf; an essential element in the development of the Self. With their own primary needs for unconditional love and attachment hanging in the balance, they focus their attention on pleasing or fixing others, particularly their caregivers, in the forlorn hope that this will make everything right. More often than not this compulsion is learned at a very early age, even before birth, and becomes a way of being in the world. If the pre-verbal child could express the underlying belief it would probably be something like, "If I could only please or fix Mommy/Daddy then she/he would be there for me and I won't die."

The incomplete Self of the parent consumes the fledgling Self of the child.

Unfortunately the child's attempts to please are often reinforced by varying degrees of success; words of praise,

No child can ever fulfill the unmet needs of a parent and the responsibility for this lies fully and solely with that parent.

occasional smiles and gentle touches embedded in brief episodes of cherished parental attention. These momentary successes are no more than leaky lifeboats on a sea of failure. For the child, the issue is survival, and every failure is fraught with desperation followed by a determination to try harder next time. Eventually the failures may be translated into beliefs that become incorporated into the child's emerging sense of Self – "I am bad, unworthy, incompetent, not doing my job." Alternatively the child who becomes highly successful in pleasing others may become attached to the image of his or her own 'goodness', creating what D. W. Winnicott referred to as a 'false self'. Thoughts, feelings and behaviors that might tarnish this image are denied and repressed into an unconscious realm that Carl Jung identified as "the shadow" – the dark side of goodness. Either way the authentic Self is pressed into the service of others. To this end, parent and child are co-conspirators in an erroneous and self-defeating belief system. Both fail to recognize that no child can ever fulfill the unmet needs of a parent and the responsibility for this lies fully and solely with that parent.

Jack Rosenberg has coined the term "agency" or more precisely, "other-agency," to identify this common theme. By this he means that the person gives up his or her own self-volition to become an agent for others. To some extent this is something most people can relate to. Some of us even become professionals. Agents can be very nice people, acutely sensitive to the needs of others and appreciated for their good deeds. If they are aware of their 'agency' habit, they know instinctively when they have given themselves away again in an attempt to please or fix another person. Given the ability to make a distinction between an act of kindness and an act of agency they can begin to address their compulsion. Dedicated agents lack such awareness. With no solid sense of Self to relinquish, they respond automatically to an unconscious or cellular message. I don't mean to imply that dedicated agents are fundamentally different from the rest of us; it really is a matter of degree. Since this topic will re-appear in subsequent discussions, I want to be clear that in using the term 'agency,' I am referring to an automatic response to an underlying belief that our place in the world is contingent upon our ability to please or fix others. For the time being I will leave it at that.

CHAPTER THREE

A Star is Born

Throughout the preceding chapter I attempted to identify the early psychological and relational influences that shape our lives prior to birth. My underlying proposition is that when we become aware of these influences we are no longer bound to repeat the patterns of the past. With a belief in our potential to take ownership of our lives, and the courage to act on our own behalf, we can move toward increasing levels of self-responsibility; the ability to respond to the world in the here and now. This isn't about changing nature; it's about being with nature. In creating the lives we want our challenge is to work with the natural order in much the same way a skilled mariner will engage wind and tide to steer a particular course. Through science we have come to see the natural order as an external reality imposed on our lives. What we have failed to recognize is that we are an integral part of that design and awareness of our internal experience is essential to our understanding of nature's way. Only when these two dimensions of reality are brought together will we recognize our place and purpose in the scheme of things and understand that when we make changes within our own lives through creative thought and purposeful action, we change all of life - past, present and future. This is the nature of interconnectedness that is as true in the world of

When we make changes within our own lives through creative thought and purposeful action, we change all of life - past, present and future.

molecular physics as it is in the flow of consciousness that links us to our ancestors, our parents, our children and future generations for eternity. My overwhelming conviction is that the time has come for us as a species to wake up, change course and take our place as conscious participants in the unfolding realm we call the universe. If we choose to remain asleep waiting for science, politics or divine intervention to see us through, the universe will incorporate whatever we have contributed and move on without us.

I have argued that the patterns that both facilitate and inhibit our potential for self-directed action are in place well before we are born. Genetics aside this is very different from traditional theories of development, at least the ones I was taught. Most of my teachers seemed to believe that we all enter this world as passive organisms waiting for genes, brains and environmental conditions to intermingle and determine what we do, who we are and what we will become – the good old tabula rasa hypothesis. I respected their scientific integrity but I was never convinced they actually believed this about themselves. To be true to their cause they would have to believe that even this opinion is no more than the outcome of their own learning histories, but such humility was never apparent.

Birth: An Indelible Memory

If we do indeed come into this world as conscious relational beings, the experience of our birth must be recognized as a pivotal point on our developmental odyssey. Within the course of nature it seems we are the initial decision makers in determining the timing of this event. When we decide the pregnancy has lasted long enough, we alert mother by increasing the flow of estrogen thereby raising the level of irritability and responsiveness of the uterine muscles. A mother who is attuned to her child responds by indicating her own state of readiness and when she is prepared for labor to begin. In other words birth, just like gestation, is a collaborative affair from the outset, a mutually choreographed event. To understand this collaboration in physiological terms it is important to recognize the nature and role of the placenta. In biology this is the only organ created by two distinct organisms, a merging of cells to form a unique system of communication that to a large extent, remains a mystery. What we do know is that if this delicate communion between mother and child is interrupted or by passed, both parties are equally disenfranchised.

However the decision is made there can be no turning back. Within the space of a few short hours, we are plunged into a life-death drama. The world we have come to know and trust is systematically shut down. She, who has always been there to nourish and nurture releases her embrace and pushes us away from our shared and sacred place. Caught up in forces beyond our control we are on our own as never before. Our bodies turn and twist in unfamiliar contortions as we struggle to unlock the resources nature has provided to take us from our protected sanctuary and out into the unknown. Our time has come and whatever we have learned from the beginning is put to the test. Whether we choose to abandon ourselves in fear, fight against the odds, or move purposefully within nature's way, our lives will never be the same again. If we learned to trust we will know our struggle is shared; we have not been deserted and She who cares will be waiting to welcome us on the other side. This is a simple faith based in experience, yet drawn from the wisdom of countless generations that went before. If we learned to stay open and receptive our senses will remain fully alive, responding to each new sensation and committing every moment to memory. If we can draw upon our own resources to overcome the obstacles and move through the fear and the pain to reconnect with our most intimate partner eye to eye, the bond will survive the ordeal. Then we will take our rightful place at the centre of our experience. This is the moment of truth, an undeniable recognition of our separateness and a reaffirmation of our interconnectedness in the new realm.

Throughout the ebb and flow of life the human Self must learn to deal with constant interruptions. For the most part we take these in our stride, pausing occasionally to lick our wounds and generate the awareness we need to take the next developmental step. If we find ourselves stuck in the mire we can always seek help to get the wheels turning again. But birth is not part of that ebb and flow; it's a once in a lifetime transformational event. The learning that takes place here, conscious or otherwise, forms the bedrock of our personal experience. This may not be readily apparent in our momentary thoughts or everyday behaviors but is revealed through the enduring characteristics and themes that play out in our lives. We are talking here about our underlying motivations and beliefs including our desire to live life to the full, our belief in our own self-volition, our level of openness and curiosity, our trust in others, and our view of the world as a friendly or hostile place. Above all the birth experience is a relational occasion that sets the course for how we will tackle life's most tantalizing developmental challenge; to establish a clear and autonomous sense of Self through relationships with others.

This is the moment of truth, an undeniable recognition of our separateness and a reaffirmation of our interconnectedness in the new realm.

Incredible as it now seems, while training to become a psychologist I was consistently told that speculations about subjective birth experiences were scientifically unfounded and developmentally irrelevant. The argument was that 'prenates' and 'neonates' are essentially senseless life forms lacking the necessary apparatus to feel, think and remember - these faculties only emerging through the first twelve months

Above all the birth experience is a relational occasion that sets the course for how we will tackle life's most tantalizing developmental challenge; to establish a clear and autonomous sense of Self through relationships with others.

of postnatal life. Even at that time I was very aware that psychoanalysts, including Sigmund Freud and Otto Rank had drawn clear links between birth experiences and subsequent mental health. According to their analytic model, repressed birth memories are stored in the unconscious and brought to light through dreams, hypnosis and therapeutic regression. Rank even went so far as to suggest that virtually all adult psychological problems, particularly those considered to be 'pathological,' could be traced back to repressed birth trauma. While it must be acknowledged that much of their clinical evidence was derived from work with adults experiencing significant psychological and psychosomatic difficulties, this in no way detracts from the conclusion that for all of us, birth is a momentous step along the developmental pathway. Yet my teachers were steadfast in their stance and resisted discussion on the topic.

Since then, thanks to the work of investigators like Nandor Fodor, Leslie LeCron, Stanislav Grof and the irrepressible David Chamberlain, we are left in do doubt that adults can, and do, remember the details of whatever took place during their birth. Within traditional academic and professional ranks these findings have been largely ignored. At one time I considered these 'experts' to be misguided but I have come to believe that theirs' is a deliberate strategic stance designed to protect their revered theories and justify their cold-hearted practices.

The importance of prenatal and birth memory is that it provides the link between these primary experiences and the awareness we need to become self-conscious and subsequently, self-directed. Since birth occurs before the development of language it is experienced as a plethora of body sensations and mental images that cannot be accurately retrieved through thought or expressed in words. In their book *Parenting from the Inside Out*, (published 2004) Daniel J. Siegal and Mary Hartzell make a useful distinction between 'implicit' and 'explicit' memory to describe how the pre-verbal brain creates particular circuits to process generalized perceptions, emotions and bodily sensations. This implicit memory forms mental models from which the infant constructs generalized characteristic patterns of perceiving and responding to the world.

Given that birth is an intense drama that occurs when we are at our most vulnerable it is more than likely some of these implicit memories will be painful and therefore, repressed. While Siegal and Hartzell are primarily concerned with neurological processes, somatic psychologists would argue that these repressed memories become physically manifested as energetic holding patterns in the body. Based largely upon the theories of the radical psychoanalyst Wilhelm Reich, somatic psychology is concerned with how the body creates its own defenses against traumatic experience by blocking the flow of energy to the areas holding the distress. Whether locked into the psyche or the body, this repressed material forms an unconscious undertow that constantly pulls us toward pre-determined ways of being in the world. Often confused with 'personality', this defensive self-defeating pattern will remain unless the original experiences can be brought into awareness and released through mental and somatic action.

Whether locked into the psyche or the body, this repressed material forms an unconscious undertow that constantly pulls us toward pre-determined ways of being in the world.

The idea that human memory involves an integration of body and mind has become widely accepted in clinical psychology and psychiatry. At the same time, many forms of psychotherapy have either acknowledged, or been directed specifically toward birth trauma and its resolution. Recognizing birth as a pre-verbal experience, the most enlightened approaches invite the client or patient to actually 're-live' rather than simply 'remember' the traumatic event. In therapeutic bodywork this re-visitation reaches beyond the brain to identify and release body memories that can then be accessed and assimilated into conscious awareness. In the early days direct hands-on manipulation of the musculature was the preferred method of treatment, but body-focused psychotherapy has become considerably more sophisticated and holistic in recent years. Nowadays many practitioners prefer to use the person's own breath as the primary vehicle for discovering and releasing the energetic memory blocks.

Of particular relevance to birthing the contributions of pioneers like William Emerson and Raymond Castellino deserve special attention. Rather than wait for difficulties to emerge later in life, these clinicians use direct energetic approaches to identify and resolve birth trauma in babies and infants. In effect they create subtle energetic shifts through which the baby re-lives the epic experiences of birth. In moments of distress, the infant receives the loving comfort and assurances of the mother who remains fully present and engaged throughout the process. Engaging the 'implicit' circuitry of the brain, the infant is able to express and move through the trauma without having to detach from the experience and repress the painful memory. This also serves to heal any damage to the mother-child bond resulting from the original experience. I can say from personal experience that while this process can be quite disturbing to observe, the subsequent reconnection between mother and child is remarkable and profoundly heart-warming.

If you're interested in the theories and practices of somatic psychotherapy, you may wish to read *Getting in Touch: The Guide to New Body-Centered Therapies*, edited by Christine Caldwell and first published in 1997. These forms of therapy are a far cry from the standard methods of traditional practice and as such, have been a target for considerable criticism if not derision, from therapists who believe that talking, modifying behavior, and pushing pills, are the only ways to go. As a graduate student I remember attending a presentation in which our most renowned faculty member used a series of silly cartoons and recorded animal noises to ridicule the work of American psychologist Arthur Janov – the man who coined the term 'primal scream' to describe the terror of the birthing infant. Presumably we were all supposed to have a good laugh before returning to our analysis of the effects of variable ratio reinforcement schedules on the behavior of laboratory rats. I was certainly amused but more by the antics of this acclaimed 'scientist' than the content of his presentation.

If my own colleagues have been slow to modify their beliefs about birth and adjust their practices accordingly, medical professionals in general have remained stubbornly resistant and aloof. While I have no quantifiable data on the subject, it seems to me that most physicians continue to regard pregnancy as a physical condition and birth as a medical event in which the mother is the 'patient' and the infant a foreign object to be removed. The most disturbing aspect of this stance is the expressed or tacit belief that babies don't feel pain – at least not like the rest of us. Much as I am horrified by this assumption I can understand why they would choose to stick to their guns. The acknowledgment of pregnancy as an emerging relationship between two sentient beings, with birth as a profound transformational experience for both parties, reduces many standard medical practices to the level of barbarism.

I could easily devote an entire chapter to the tragic implications of modern medical birthing practices but David Chamberlain has already done this with compelling conviction and clarity. In his words, "In the last hundred years, scientific authorities robbed babies of their cries by calling them 'echoes' or 'random sound'; robbed them of their smiles by calling them 'gas'; robbed them of their memories by calling them 'fantasies'; and robbed them of their pain by calling it a 'reflex'" (p. 145a).

> *Most physicians continue to regard pregnancy as a physical condition and birth as a medical event in which the mother is the 'patient' and the infant a foreign object to be removed.*

There can be no question that modern technology has provided us with incredible insights into the physiology of birthing along with many sophisticated techniques for ensuring the physical well being of mother and child. The unfortunate irony is that the application of this technology so often creates the very distress it was designed to ameliorate. The problem is not so much in the technology as in the attitude of the technicians. At the broadest level this is reflected in the refusal to recognize the psychological significance of the birth experience – for both mother and child. Obstetrician and gynecologist Paul Brenner in his inspirational little book, *Life is a Shared Creation*, eloquently express this problem:

> *It has become clear to me that the one aspect that traditional Western medicine has neglected in its quest for technical immortality is the biopsychosocial model of the patient. Technology's battle against death can destroy human dignity in the quest for survival. The fear of death often distracts us from our greater fear of life. Modern medicine tends to overlook the empirical fact that life is more than living. (p.131).*

Later he writes:

> *The rite of birth is no more than a momentous point in human time that is experienced and shared by all. It is as if life speaks once again: "Play it again. Travel on the laser of life. Be willing to accept the path of love as well as the path of pain, each is your teacher. Have no fear, you can't help but learn. That's why you're here!" The babe cries, "But what am I here to learn?" Life softly replies, "To answer your own questions and to share your answers with me." (p. 135).*

Brenner's delightful blend of medicine, psychology and mysticism connects the parts to the whole without blame or incrimination but this is far removed from the disconnected myopic world of the stereotypical hospital birthing room.

Given what we now know it's easy to take arms against the medical profession, but physicians are not the enemy. On the contrary most are dedicated professionals whose primary objective is to repair our bodies, cure our diseases and preserve our lives. I for one admire their achievements and remain eternally grateful for their efforts. I am certainly not suggesting they should stay out of the birthing room; my plea is for them to broaden their perspective and recognize their critical role in an unfolding human drama that is the very essence of our developmental journey. I realize there may be perfectly valid medical reasons for intervening in the process. What I ask is that such interruptions be recognized and that every effort made to ensure that reconnection occurs as soon as possible afterwards. With this in mind I invite physicians to consider the documented and potential psychological impact of their routine birthing practices on the mother, the child and their emerging relationship.

In highlighting my concerns I wish I could refer to an impressive body of 'scientific' studies but, unfortunately, medical and psychological researchers in general have chosen to avoid investigating this absolutely fundamental episode in human development. In my opinion the reasons for this 'oversight' are essentially political and financial. As it stands the task has been left to a relatively small group of self-supporting pioneers in the field of pre-and-perinatal psychology who continue to promote primal health research as a legitimate epidemiological avenue of enquiry.

Appropriate to the nature of the phenomena under investigation, their findings offer a rich combination of empirical, clinical and anecdotal material. In the following examples I will certainly draw upon this body of work, but much of what I have to say is 'painfully' obvious. I don't need a meteorologist to tell me when it's raining.

> *I invite physicians to consider the documented and potential psychological impact of their routine birthing practices on the mother, the child and their emerging relationship.*

The Drug Culture

The most common feature of modern birthing is undoubtedly the use of drugs. In her book *Unassisted Childhood*, published in 1994, Laura Shanley reported that, in North America, analgesia, anesthesia and epidurals (which contain the same anesthesia administered intravenously) are routinely administered in over 80% of hospital births. Although usually administered to the mother, these drugs find their way into the delicate systems of the baby with harmful physical consequences. Over thirty years ago researchers such as Doris Haire and W. F. Windle were already warning us about the relationship between obstetrical medication and brain damage, retardation and learning disabilities. Curiously enough there has been little systematic follow-up to these studies. When it comes to the psychological impact of these drugs the 'scientific' evidence is even more scant. Yet based upon thirty years of research and clinical practice reported in his publication *Birth Trauma: The Psychological Effects of Obstetrical Interventions*, psychologist William Emerson firmly concludes: "the most frequent obstetrical intervention, the use of anesthetics, may be one of the most harmful, physically and psychologically." (p.49). Do we really need statistical evidence to arouse our concerns? With particular reference to the themes of the preceding chapters, I would suggest that the following concerns are either self-evident or at least worthy of very serious consideration.

The rationale for the routine use of anesthesia is that they ameliorate the pain of the mother; generally a respected medical objective. Unfortunately, one physical 'side effect' is that these pain blockers render both mother and child less able to push creating a condition known as 'failure to progress'. The obstetrical response is usually a call for additional forms of intervention and the medical snowball begins to roll. The physical outcomes are a major concern, but what about the psychological implications of mother's medicated condition? Stated bluntly, numbed out pain means numbed-out awareness. This means that mother's state of presence - her conscious and energetic availability to her birthing partner - is compromised during this most critical transformation in their emerging relationship. This constitutes abandonment at the most primal level. It also means that she loses her place as co-director in the drama leaving the child to struggle on alone. If both parties are equally anesthetized they share a common state of helplessness at a time when the foundations of empowerment and self-efficacy are being established.

William Emerson uses the term 'anesthesia shock' to describe the sudden and unexpected physiological and psychological impact of this medication. He contends that these drugs overwhelm the sensory, motor, emotional and cognitive systems of birthing babies. The child's subjective experience is one of terror

> *If both parties are equally anesthetized they share a common state of helplessness at a time when the foundations of empowerment and self-efficacy are being established.*

followed by a loss of awareness and energy, giving rise to a sense of being out of control. Developmentally these interruptions may well occur at a critical moment in the emergence of the infant's sense of self-efficacy - "I was doing fine; I could have done it on my own." Within the mother-child relationship such experiences are passed back and forth through the placental interface. In other words, the learning is mutual and debilitating on both sides.

Emerson and his colleagues have much to say about how these birthing experiences are played out in later life - this matter will be explored in some detail later. My intention here is to consider what might be taking place through the birthing process. Questions we might ask include: "What are the likely effects of mother's non-presence on the primal relationship, the essential bond? What are the implications of her lack of participation in this primal event? What does the child learn at the most basic or cellular level about his or her efficacy in the strange new world? How does the child come to terms with the fear of abandonment, of being alone in the struggle between life and death? In what ways do these formative experiences influence subsequent development?" Of course we have few 'scientific' answers to such questions but if basic empathy and commonsense are allowed to prevail, we must surely take them very seriously. Through research conducted with animals, it has been clearly demonstrated that anesthesia has a profound effect on maternal behavior often culminating in neglect and rejection of the offspring. While the effect on humans might be more complex, why would we not expect the same basic outcome?

Returning to the matter of maternal pain during birth, I realize I am stepping into contentious territory. It may be fine to talk philosophically about pain and anguish as essential human experiences but establishing their place in the birthing process raises all kinds of political, moral and gender based issues. Many commentators, admittedly most of them males, have argued that birthing is a primal preparation for life and the physical distress of mother and child is a necessary part of nature's prescription. Ironically these include some of the most prominent proponents of 'natural' or 'gentle' birthing, such as French obstetrician Frederick Leboyer, author of *Birth Without Violence* and American Robert Bradley, the pioneer of 'husband-coached childbirth'. Leboyer makes his point thus:

> *With its heart bursting, the infant sinks into hell...the mother is driving it out. At the same time, she is holding it in, preventing its passage. It is she who is the enemy. She who stands between the child and life. Only one of them can prevail. It is mortal combat ... not satisfied with crushing, the monster (mother) twists in its refinement of cruelty. (Mitford p.65).*

At its ontological core this position suggests that the fluctuation of synergy and antagonism between mother and child becomes an embodiment of the most deeply rooted dichotomies of the Self – connection and conflict, love and hate, pain and pleasure, abandonment and invasion, life and death. The juxtaposition of these experiences is both a preparation for life and a metaphor for human existence. Their union is the process of life itself returning into wholeness. Life without pain is not only impossible but also undesirable. If this sounds overly abstract and philosophical it is interesting to note that the same antagonistic dynamic is also taking place at the biological level. Throughout birthing, mother and child release increased levels of adrenaline associated with 'fight and flight,' and oxytocin, associated with altruism and love. According to Michael Odent, Director of the Primal Health Research Centre in London, the delicate balance between these two hormones is an integral if not essential, ingredient in the birthing of all mammals.

Alternatively we have the argument that much of the pain experienced during birth is a direct or indirect consequence of tension brought on by the mother's fears, before and during the birthing process. The 'natural childbirth' movement, pioneered by English obstetrician Grantly Dick-Read in the 1930's, has continued to promote prenatal education along with techniques of 'release' breathing, relaxation and meditation. While these approaches have been widely adopted as preparatory measures across the developed world, medical

Life without pain is not only impossible but also undesirable.

birthing practices continue to be anything but 'natural'. Fear created by intrusive procedures and pain numbed out by drugs is still the order of the day when the medics move in and the *real* work begins. It seems that only in exceptional and privileged circumstances is birth expected to be a potentially fulfilling and joyful experience. In her book *The American Way of Birth*, Jessica Mitford offers a fascinating and disturbing analysis of the political, legal and economic forces that operate to ensure that the medical status quo is rigidly maintained. She observes, "there seems to be no doubt that for the affluent, and those with large, inclusive health insurance policies, hospital birth today can be a highly enjoyable experience" (p.?). This concern lies beyond the parameters of the present discussion. When it comes to the matter at hand I settle for the middle ground by suggesting that distress during birth is both natural and circumstantial. From this perspective the intention should be to offer support through the former and minimize the impact of the latter. Unfortunately modern birthing practices are inclined to create the exact opposite.

Wherever possible, it is the mother who should decide how she wishes to give birth. My only concern is that such decisions should be made with full awareness, based upon an understanding of all available options and the potential consequences for both herself and her unborn child.

Beyond the rigidity of the medical professions, much of the controversy surrounding the use of drugs to control pain during birthing has been focused upon the mother and argued within the context of 'women's rights'. In effect this debate has added more confusion than clarity to the issue. In my opinion, wherever possible, it is the mother who should decide how she wishes to give birth. My only concern is that such decisions should be made with full awareness, based upon an understanding of all available options and the potential consequences for both herself and her unborn child. In this she is the expert with access to generations of accumulated wisdom and anything that serves to diminish that awareness or take away her autonomy, compromises the delicate balance of nature's design. Is it possible that this wisdom has been distorted by the stories and images of distress created by medical beliefs and practices? Would women make different choices if they anticipated birthing as a potentially joyful experience? What difference would it make if mothers were encouraged to relate to their unborn children as sentient beings and partners throughout the pregnancy? My proposition is that with such awareness and support, most women would make decisions in the best interests of themselves and their child. This is very different from advocating a woman's right to a pain-free birth.

I have already alluded to the fact that obstetrical interventions in the birthing process tend to snowball. Where anesthesia diminish the ability of mother and child to push, and 'failure to progress' becomes a concern, other drugs are used to counteract the problem – typically Pitocin. This drug intensifies the contractions creating increased pain, which in turn leads to the administration of more anesthesia or analgesia. This cycle can quickly escalate to bring about more intrusive means of augmentation or induction through the use of surgical instruments, suction and cesarean surgery. Clinical evidence suggests that the psychological effects of Pitocin often reappear later in life as a sense of being pushed and harassed, leading to feelings of paranoia and persecution. According to William Emerson, when this drug is used to augment or induce delivery it serves to operate as "a reinforcement of inadequacy, initially experienced during induction" (p.73). If Emerson is correct then we have every reason to be concerned about the effects of such drugs on the subsequent development of self-efficacy and personal autonomy. When it comes to the more direct physical implications we are only just beginning to understand the immediate impact of multiple obstetric medications on the fragile fetal brain, although the potential long-term effects, such as learning disabilities and drug addiction, are slowly coming to light.

In most cases the use of Pitocin requires electronic fetal monitoring. By restricting the mother's ability to move this technology increases the likelihood of extended labor and thereby, 'failure to progress'. This in turn, may lead to particularly intrusive and painful monitoring procedures, including the screwing of electrodes in the baby's skull while still in the birth canal. All this is designed to determine the level of 'fetal distress'; a common rationale for additional augmentation and induction interventions. And so the medical machine rolls on, creating what it purports to ameliorate. There is no doubt that electronic fetal monitoring. a proud symbol of modern technology is one of the major reasons for the dramatic increase in cesarean births over the past thirty years. Again the most significant issue is not the machine itself but the attitudes of those who operate it. If physicians used this technology to experience their innate connection to the birthing child, rather than strive for a problem free delivery, perhaps they would be more willing to let nature take its course. By focusing upon the mother's ability to give birth rather than their own methods for delivering birth, they might come to see themselves as humble participants in this momentous transformational event. Meanwhile they could make use of their machines to observe the impact of their presence and behavior on the child. Such research would be both fascinating and invaluable.

If physicians used this technology to experience their innate connection to the birthing child, rather than strive for a problem free delivery, perhaps they would be more willing to let nature take its course.

We Have the Technology

I realize there will always be occasions when the course of nature threatens life and medical intervention is clearly indicated. I also realize this is a time when the attending medics have more to think about than their own existential issues. This is also a time when mothers and babies are most vulnerable and what occurs will likely have substantial developmental implications. The immediate preservation of life may be the number one priority but sensitivity to the experience of mother and child, along with recognition that these intrusive interruptions will need to be addressed later, must surely be part of the equation. The use of surgical instruments, fetal heart monitors, respirators and vacuum extractors are all potentially damaging to the child's physical, mental and emotional development. The failure to recognize these risks is simply unacceptable. In the words of David Chamberlain, "Everyone who deals with babies will have to cope with the fact that sentience and consciousness are permanent aspects of the human psyche. There are no free periods at the beginning of life when violent treatment can be offered babies in the name of science, even 'for their own good'" (p.115a). To this I would like to add that the same principle applies at the other end of the life-span.

On the brighter side there are some indications that physicians do respond favorably to feedback when it is generated within their own medical domain. A good example is the virtual elimination of 'forceps delivery' after countless studies had documented the hazards of this procedure and lawyers began to move in for the kill. Advances in psychobiology, neurochemistry and endocrinology, along with the technology of ultrasound and intrauterine photography have made it increasingly possible to observe and assess an infant's sensitivity and responsiveness through gestation and birth. Hopefully this 'objective' evidence will eventually serve to open the eyes, ears and hearts of those who monitor pregnancies and facilitate deliveries. Around the world physicians have been voicing their objections to the medical circumcision of newborns on the grounds that it is both painful and unnecessary. Even more encouraging are the reports of doctors who are electing to replace or augment mechanical devices with the most basic form of communication – human touch. Massage and the gentle manipulation of an infant lodged in the birth canal offers a simple alternative to technology. In one report doctors described their success in actually 'talking' babies out of breach positions to complete otherwise unassisted deliveries. It's interesting to note that the major obstacle they had to overcome was the embarrassment they experienced in talking to a fetus. But taken together these are still only glimmers of a more humane future in the birthing business.

Perhaps the most significant shift in birthing practices over the past forty years has been the dramatic escalation of cesarean deliveries, particularly in the developed world. If present trends continue the percentage of cesarean births will pass the fifty-per-cent level within the next decade. Once considered to be an emergency measure, technology has enhanced the safety and efficiency of this procedure to the point where it is now commonplace and the method of choice for increasing numbers of women and their medical advisors. While we might understand why a mother would choose to avoid the stress and unpredictability of labour, the bypassing of the birthing process for the sake of convenience has many developmental and relational implications; not only for mother and child, but for society in general.

Given all I have said thus far about the crucial nature of prenatal and perinatal learning, my own thoughts about cesarean delivery should be no surprise. In my view this trend represents the handing over of human birth to the medical profession, hook, line and sinker. In making this choice women sacrifice their own autonomy and thereby deny their children the opportunity to come into this world under their own steam. I could go on a rant about the psychological implications in terms of self-efficacy, locus of control, intrinsic motivation, self-esteem, empathy, relational autonomy etc., but this hardly seems necessary. The overall effect is that both mother and child are equally debilitated, and unless some remedial action is taken after the surgery, they will spend the rest of their lives searching elsewhere for the missing piece. I am reminded of a simple anecdote attributed to Confucius:

> One day, a small opening appeared in a cocoon. A man watched the butterfly for several hours as it struggled to force its body through that little hole. Then it seemed to stop making progress. It appeared as if it had gotten as far as is could, and could go no further. So the man decided to help the butterfly: he took a pair of scissors and opened the cocoon. The butterfly emerged easily. But it had a withered body, it was tiny with shriveled wings. The man continued to watch because he expected that, at any moment, the wings would open, enlarge and expand, to be able to support the butterfly's body and become firm. Neither happened! In fact, the butterfly spent the rest of its life crawling around with its withered body and shriveled wings. It never was able to fly. What the man in his kindness and his good will did not understand was that the restricting cocoon and the struggle required by the butterfly through the tiny opening were God's way of forcing fluid from the body and into the wings, so that it would be ready for flight once it achieved its freedom. Sometimes, struggles are exactly what we need in our life. If God allowed us to go through life without any obstacles, it would cripple us. We would never be as strong as we could have been ... never able to fly.

I can only wonder about the future of a society in which this fundamental phase of human development is surgically removed and where large segments of the population willingly place their lives in the hands of those who promise a painless passage to the Promised Land. The one thing we can be sure of is that the beneficiaries of this transaction are not about to investigate our inability to fly.

Unless there is a dramatic shift in attitude such investigation will be left to a handful of renegade researchers whose findings will continue to receive little attention in the medical establishment and the public media. So far such research strongly indicates that women who give birth by cesarean section exhibit significantly lower levels of perceived control and higher levels of depression and physiological distress. Epidemiological data accumulated by Michael Odent and his colleagues at the Primal Health Research Centre, confirm that we have every reason to be perturbed about the effects of such intrusive birthing procedures on the subsequent development of the child. Documented correlations between these practices and the incidence of asthma, anorexia nervosa, suicide, learning disability, self-esteem, autism and juvenile criminality, are just some of the findings that await further investigation. If nothing else these studies have posed many unanswered questions about the relationship between the birth experience and physical and psychological health.

Again I want to emphasize that before or during labor, there may be perfectly valid reasons to opt for a cesarean delivery. All I ask is that the vaginal birth be reconsidered and recognized as the preferred option in the best interests of both mother and child and that the developmental implications of obstetric

I believe it is now possible to bring together the marvels of modern technology with the humanistic methods developed by birth-trauma clinicians.

interventions be carefully assessed and addressed. My hope is that decisions will be made by sensitive and well informed human beings. Given such conditions I believe it is now possible to bring together the marvels of modern technology with the humanistic methods developed by birth-trauma clinicians. Where the mother is not able to be fully present for the delivery, her role may be temporarily delegated to someone whose sole responsibility is to 'be there' for her child until she is able to reconnect and re-establish the bond that is so essential for both of their lives. The overarching objective should be to ensure that mother and child will have the opportunity to experience birth as a meaningful and pivotal moment; both in their individual lives and their emerging relationship.

All this implies that what happens before and during birth is inextricably linked to what occurs immediately afterwards. As Paul Brenner sees it:

> *The delivery is completed as the newborn unfolds like a flower from a contracted to an extended state and takes its first breath of freedom – deliverance. This a moment to be cheered with same emotions and sense of collective experience the world felt when Neil Armstrong took his first step on the moon – a step for all human kind. The child is a voyager from space and deserves that same welcome (p.134).*

So what kind of welcome awaits the traveler in the modern hospital birthing room? Well the chances are that the birthing partner will be lying in a drugged out state while an emotionally sterile welcoming committee hovers overhead. From the moment of 'crowning' to the clamping and severance of the umbilicus, the masked and muffled team goes about its work, far too involved with protocols to be loving and rejoicing. Surrounded by bright lights, buzzing machines and cold metallic objects the task is not to connect with another human being but to ensure 'its' successful passage through the birth canal and evaluate 'its' physical condition according to something called the "Apgar" scale. For this purpose the newcomer may be grasped in the gloved hands of strangers, suspended upside down, slapped, cleansed with stinging antiseptic solutions, weighed, stretched out and measured - the first 'human' touch. Whatever the procedure it's highly unlikely that any recognition will be given to the fact that newborns are fully aware of their own internal sensations and what is taking place around them. How different this might be if those in charge chose to look through the lens offered by David Chamberlain:

> *The view of life presented by babies at birth is an intriguing and mystical one of complete persons in little bodies knowing many things: they are frustrated that they cannot yet make their bodies work the way they'd like; they know what they need and whom they can trust; they evaluate the 'motivations' of doctors; they perceive the psychological flaws in standard medical births; they point out virtues or weaknesses of parents; and they recognize the special needs of their siblings (p.87a).*

One of the paradoxical peculiarities of medical practice is that the more serious the perceived problem, the less the concern for the sufferer. This is particularly evident in 'high-risk' situations where the patient's injury or disease becomes the sole focus of attention, and the person is regarded as a 'body-in-crisis'. This is what Paul Brenner is alluding to when he talks about destroying human dignity in the quest for survival. In western medicine this might be considered rational and justifiable, but there are other medical traditions in which the 'relationship' between doctor and patient is seen to be an essential ingredient in surgery, treatment and healing – even in the direst circumstances. I would suggest when it comes to birthing, this model is infinitely superior, and particularly when both mother and child are acknowledged as identified 'patients'. Unfortunately, the technological world remains resistant, and nowhere is this more readily apparent than in the case of the most vulnerable babies transferred to neonatal intensive care.

At the broadest level we can only theorize about a possible connection between violent births and violence in society at large, but it's a compelling idea.

Sometimes referred to as a "Theatre of Violence" or "man made womb", the NICU is a paragon of modern technology in which only the technicians have the knowledge to decide and authority to act. In this brightly lit and frequently chaotic laboratory, high-risk babies are immobilized and subjected to constant intrusions, most of them painful. Anxious parents are kept at a distance while the new life hangs in the balance. It is difficult to imagine how a newborn might be responding to this first experience of life on the outside, but can there be any doubt that even if the baby survives the ordeal physically, the emotional and psychological impact will be horrendous? There have been many questions raised about procedures used in the NICU, but my concern here is with what happens when the child is discharged back to the family if the psychological damage is not recognized and addressed. At the broadest level we can only theorize about a possible connection between violent births and violence in society at large, but it's a compelling idea.

Studies conducted by William Emerson and others have already shown that over half the children subjected to NICU procedures exhibit subsequent psychiatric problems, but this may be only the tip of the iceberg. Children who survive and appear 'normal' from a medical perspective will almost certainly carry the trauma into their lives. Unless this is understood the chances are that their subsequent developmental or psychological difficulties will be attributed to some hypothetical 'disorder' and treated accordingly. This problem is by no means limited to NICU alumni.

Relational Birthing

The birthing environment is the newborn's first direct encounter with the external world of human relationships. The child's concern is not only with each individual in attendance but also with the relationships among them. Some attendees are already 'known' and their sudden appearance as external beings is a monumental shift the infant psyche must accommodate. There are also 'known' relationships. Of course mother is by far the most significant, and the preservation of this bond is a need that transcends all others. But there may also be father or mother's partner, who has become increasingly familiar throughout the pregnancy. Since the parental relationship is an extension of the primary bond, I particularly like Paul Brenner's suggestion that "the integration and unification of mother, father, and child, may take place when the father's hands are allowed to assist in the birth process and cradle the newborn" (p.132). There may be siblings whose excitement and curiosity about the little one in mother's belly are already deeply embedded in the newcomer's experience. Ideally there will be grandparents, particularly Grandma who represents the maternal link to past generations. And there may be others, relatives and friends who form the network of relationships and stand ready to welcome another life into the fold. Then finally, there are the strangers, the unknown figures performing the rituals of their own agenda. Their moment may

There is no doubt in my mind that our earliest fears of abandonment and invasion create the foundation for all subsequent relationships.

be fleeting but their impact can be monumental.

The people and the circumstances may vary but whatever the child perceives creates a blueprint of how the world works, and whatever he or she senses from others is internalized for future reference. If the child feels welcomed with joy and love, the ingenuous Self sets out on the human journey assured of connection and full of optimism. If mother is absent physically or energetically, and if others are distant, cold, or otherwise preoccupied, the abandoned Self must face the world alone, desperate for survival. Alternatively if the infant is besieged by painful intrusions or inundated by the actions of others the child recoils as a protection from further invasion. Either way, if body and mind are one, and Bruce Lipton is correct, this fear response must apply to every aspect of the infant's being, including the complex system we call the Self.

While you might question Otto Rank's belief that birth trauma lies at the root of most mental health problems, there is no doubt in my mind that our earliest fears of abandonment and invasion create the foundation for all subsequent relationships. The interplay between these two primary sources of anxiety will become more apparent as we move along the developmental continuum into early childhood. Meanwhile you may wish to examine how your own needs for closeness and separation have influenced your life and how they play out in your current relationships. If this sparks your curiosity, you might want to trace this pattern back to your earliest experiences within your family of origin. When it comes to understanding ourselves, I will take subjective validation over scientific verification any day.

It is true that our understanding of what a child subjectively experiences and learns during birth remains speculative. However, given all the evidence – objective, subjective and intuitive – I can find absolutely no justification other than strategic denial, for the assertion that this event is psychologically insignificant. If professionals who maintain this stance were to open up the curiosity of their minds and the humanity in their hearts, they would surely move beyond their view of the newborn as an object and reconsider their birthing practices.

The general consensus among prenatal and perinatal researchers is that very few babies come into the world without significant distress. Emerson himself suspects that forty five percent of newborns experience birth trauma to the degree that they require some form of specialized treatment. Unfortunately the indicators, or symptoms, are rarely recognized because they are considered by physicians and parents to be 'normal'. For example, two to six hours of infant crying is generally considered to be within the normal range, yet babies assessed to be free of birth trauma cry for an average of only twenty minutes a day, essentially as a means of communicating their immediate needs.

Babies assessed to be free of birth trauma cry for an average of only twenty minutes a day, essentially as a means of communicating their immediate needs.

Without further elaboration I can only hope I have presented enough information to support my contention that the time has come for a major shift in our cultural attitudes toward birth, along with an immediate review and revision of current birthing practices. If you're not convinced, I can only assume that, for you, the universe is unfolding as it should and that our survival as a species has little to do with human relationships. In this case, I will acknowledge your position and move on. Consider first, a true story, kindly contributed by my partner Judith.

The Case of a Mother who 'Just Knew'

In the summer of 1997 my friend Janice, a midwife and doula working in our local community, asked me to see a thirty-four year old woman who was preparing to give birth to her third (and last) child. For 'medical reasons' her other two children had been delivered by cesarean section and her doctor was convinced that the same procedure should be followed. Heidi became distressed to the point where a psychiatrist was consulted and anti-depressive medications were being seriously considered. Worried about the implications, Janice called me for a psychological opinion.

When I asked Heidi about her desire for a vaginal birth, she placed a hand on her belly. "I just want to be with this one all the way," she said. She went on to tell me how much she loved her two daughters but always felt they had come into the world without her. She wanted me to know this wasn't about feeling guilty but about her own need to experience motherhood "to the full." Afraid to challenge her doctor's authority she decided to engage a midwife in the hope that someone would be on her side. She trusted Janice but after every medical check up, she came away feeling helpless and depressed. She looked at me through her tears. "I can do this,- I know I can," she sobbed. "This is my last chance and I've made a promise I just can't break."

With Heidi's permission Janice and I discussed the matter with the physician, and he agreed to back off from the pre-planned cesarean. He made it clear however, that this was still his recommendation and would revert to this option if necessary. With his support Heidi, Janice and I agreed to work together in the weeks prior to the anticipated event. Under our instruction Heidi became a dedicated student of mindful meditation, release breathing, somatic awareness, creative imagery and a host of rituals and practices Janice had collected over the years. She even suspended a macramé sling from a tree in the woods for Heidi to practice various pelvic movements and positions. It was serious business but there was also laughter – sometimes the deep belly laughter of women in the wild and sometimes the light-headed giggling of mischievous schoolgirls. As the days passed Heidi's depression gave way to a spirited optimism and her whole demeanor changed dramatically. She loved it when her husband Carl watched her bathe and commented, "You are so beautiful. You're not only growing, you're glowing."

On the afternoon when the first signs of labor came, I went over to Heidi's house to find the family in a state of eager anticipation. "It's as crazy as Christmas around here," Carl announced as he and Janice gathered the 'necessities' together while the two girls hovered in the background struggling to contain their excitement. Heidi remained seated on the sofa but raised her arms for a hug as I came through the door. "Welcome to the Madhouse," she said, with a smile. "Thanks for the invitation," I whispered, "I could use some madness."

I will never forget the trip to the hospital in the family 'chariot' – six of us crammed together in an old station wagon teetering on that nebulous edge between excitement and anxiety. On one hand, I felt so blessed and privileged to be included in this family occasion. On the other was the uncertainty of what was yet to come and my own part in the proceedings. Our agreement was that Janice would be there for Heidi and I would be ready to welcome the baby should anything interrupt mother's full engagement. A few days earlier when I asked Janice for specific instructions, all she said was, "Just stop being a psychologist for a couple of hours and you'll know exactly what to do." It made sense at the time.

When we arrived Heidi hugged and kissed her two girls who were returning home with a neighbor to await further instructions. As promised, each was allowed to cup her hands on mother's belly and whisper a 'secret' message to their new brother before climbing back into the car. The ritual over, Janice led us through the maternity section to the assigned birthing room. She seemed so full of confidence as she helped Heidi, Carl and myself with our preparations and introduced us to the two attending nurses. I've always disliked hospitals for the same reason I dislike law courts – something about feeling inadequate and judged. This time it was different. We were there for a purpose, joined in spirit with the strength to see it through. All I had to do was to be there.

By the time the physician arrived, Heidi was already on her back, practicing long deep belly breaths. "She's going to need time," Janice told him, "we don't want to rush this one." The doctor glanced at the wall clock – it was 3.30 in the afternoon. "Well, we'll see," he said. "Let's take a look at what's going on here." As he moved in to make his examination, Heidi's breathing immediately became shallow, barely noticeable. My own body tightened. Janice looked at me and shook her head. "We have a problem," she whispered. Upon completion the doctor came over to where we were standing. "Dilation is marginal," he told us. "You may be expecting too much." Janice placed a hand on his shoulder. "Expect the best but be prepared for anything less," she said. "My sentiments exactly," said the doctor before turning to one of the nurses. "Can we get this monitor hooked-up and have the anesthetist on standby?" Janice returned to the cause. "Well, there's not much happening, so why don't we continue with the breathing and I'll let you know if anything changes?" He hesitated for a moment. "I'll be on the third floor. Use my buzzer at 714."

Listening to their conversation I felt my body tighten as I recalled the birth of my own daughter – a terrifying and painful event in which I found myself semi-conscious, struggling to follow the instructions of distant voices. That same feeling of helplessness swept over me. I wondered if the time we had spent with Heidi in her cozy living room and the magical woods around her house would turn out to be nothing more than a romantic illusion, a joyful prelude to inevitable distress. Feeling ashamed of my self-indulgence and doubts, I looked over at Janice hoping she hadn't noticed my temporary absence. True to form our dedicated midwife had already returned to her duties.

Back in charge of operations, she moved over to the table and took Heidi's hand. "Your buddies are all here, including Carl," she said quietly. "Another deep breath, right down into the belly. Yea…that's great. You know everything you need to know and have everything you need for the adventure. This is your time and we'll be with you all the way." She bent over and kissed Heidi on the cheek. "There isn't anything you have to do for me, or for anybody else around here… we're all just fine."

I had no idea how tight my body really was until I heard these words. With one involuntary breath, my shoulders let go and the knot in my stomach dissolved. Was this what I needed to hear all those years ago - a simple affirmation of my own volition, my own 'rightness.' I was about to chastise myself again when I noticed that Heidi had taken a similar breath and we were now breathing to the same rhythm. Perhaps it wasn't self-indulgence after all. Perhaps we were just two women in communion, sharing an experience across time and space - a strange idea that I still don't fully understand. Yet Janice seemed to be tuned into the same channel. "Great," she said, "everybody breathe, let's all breathe together. You lead Heidi."

From our places around the birthing table, we listened to Janice's progress reports. "Dilation has moved from two to four centimeters," she told us, as we continued to focus our attention on the rise and fall of Heidi's belly. "No need to rush here, everything's just as it should be." As in a dream I lost all sense of time. There was nothing that separated one moment from the next. Even our breathing seemed to blend into a symphonic flow with Heidi setting the tempo. It was as if we had all surrendered ourselves to some other imperative.

The doctor returned as a stranger, if not an intruder. He glanced at the clock on the wall. It was ten to six. Janice moved away from where she had been hovering between Heidi's knees, granting him access to his patient. He looked at the monitor and moved in for a closer examination, placing his stethoscope on Heidi's belly. With the assistance of one of the nurses, another monitoring device, a tocodynamometer, was strapped to her lower abdomen. We could all see and probably feel, the effect on the patient. Her breathing became locked into her chest and her body stiffened. We were back in the hospital, attending to protocols and anxiously awaiting outcomes. I moved to Janice's side and put my arm around her waist. She smiled and nodded but I could see the concern in her face. Finally the physician came over and pulled off his mask and gloves. "Well, there don't appear to be any serious complications, but it's slow, very slow. There's certainly dilation but we should be crowning and contracting by now. I think a mild induction might be in the best interest of mother and child at this point." Janice thought for a moment. "Can we talk outside for a couple minutes?" "Yes, of course." When they left I went over to make contact with Heidi. She tried to smile but her normally soft and expressive face was rigid and non-compliant. I held out my hand and she grasped it instantly. "Our plan isn't going to work is it?" she asked. "Nothing has changed so far," I told her. "Janice is talking to your doctor now. Meanwhile, some breathing might help all of us."

Janice returned alone. After a brief chat with Carl, she came to share the good news. "Okay, check-out time has been extended folks, let's get the show back on the road. EVERYBODY BREATHE!" The nurses laughed, Carl beamed and Heidi bless her heart, was finally able to smile.

It was a busy evening. Janice arranged for Heidi to be unhooked from the machines and had her walking slowly around the room in a matter of minutes. Then we three 'women of the wild woods' bundled ourselves together, ambled down the long hospital corridor and out into the gentle silence of the night. We sang softly, whispered our beloved chants, talked to the bushes and giggled just as before. It took Janice's concern for hospital etiquette to keep us appropriate and contained. We were strolling across a deserted parking lot when the contractions started in earnest. Heidi was joking about giving birth in a tree sling at the time. Arm in arm, our trek back to the birthing room was unhurried but definitely purposeful. It was eleven-twenty when we finally arrived.

The early going was full of stops and starts but the doctor, fresh from six hours of uninterrupted sleep, seemed quite prepared to allow nature to take its course. Meanwhile Janice remained close at her friend's side, quietly assuring and gently encouraging. I sat next to Carl my arm around his shoulders, as we waited for information and instructions from the inner circle. It was almost four in the morning when Heidi's cervix fully dilated and the baby's head appeared. There were some tense moments during his short journey down the birth canal and the physician decided to perform a last minute episiotomy. Respecting Heidi's wishes the local anesthetic employed for this procedure was the only drug used throughout.

I have tried many times to describe my experience of witnessing the birth of another human being, but my words could never capture that incredible moment when a new life first appears. To be fully present, allowing all the senses to perceive and the emotions to respond is an act of sublime faith – a surrender to our own Creation. I can understand why medical people might choose to cut themselves off from such intensity and focus on the mechanics of cutting cords and delivering placentas. When Heidi's baby finally eased himself into the world my heart sang out and every fiber of my being seemed to come alive. I needed no instructions. I turned to Carl who was standing beside me. "He's here, Carl. Your son has arrived. Just look at him…isn't he absolutely beautiful?" As I looked into the father's tear-filled eyes, I knew that this baby had come to the right place at the right time. "And so are you," I added.

Once the cord had been clamped and cut, the baby was handed over to the nurses and the customary medical protocols were performed with commendable efficiency. Janice then carefully removed the hospital wrap and placed the naked infant beneath mother's breasts – skin-to-skin, belly-to-belly. Janice beckoned for Carl to join her and pointed for me to move to the other side of the table. The baby was crying, soft gentle whimpers, arms and legs stretching and recoiling as if to sense out the strange new world. We watched and waited, but Heidi made no move. With the bed now raised into a semi-upright position, she looked down on her new son like someone observing a distant and unbelievable event. After a few moments, Janice took hold of Heidi's elbows and cradling the baby between his mother's arms, lifted him gently until he was nestled securely in the valley of her breasts. Resting on his back, his eyes wide open, he fixed his attention on the face of the women who had brought him to this place. She continued to stare back at him, but her face seemed strangely blank and lifeless.

There is a precious moment of re-connection between a mother and her newborn child known simply as 'the gaze'. This is an energetic and some would say spiritual, reunion of fellow travelers who have moved cautiously, and sometimes painfully, through the unknown to find themselves on the other side, transformed and embodied in another realm. For the mother this is an undeniable recognition of separateness – a visual confirmation that another human being has inhabited her body. Looking into the mother's eyes, the child becomes aware of himself or herself in the world for the very first time. If mother is there to acknowledge the newcomer, the child receives the messages that will lay the foundation for being – "I am here. I exist and I am welcome here. What I knew on the inside is here on the outside. I am not alone. I am valued – I am loved. My new life is confirmed and assured." The gaze contains the seeds for all that is to follow.

It was my job to be there for Heidi's baby. I sensed something was missing and felt a deep sadness in my heart when his face crinkled up, his forehead red and furrowed. When he began to cry, I wanted to cry with him but instead of baby tears there were adult words. "That was a hard journey," I said softly. "But now you're here and it's all over. Your mother is here for you, just as she has always been. You are so special, so wonderful and so welcome." His face relaxed and the crying subsided. Then Heidi took over, hesitatingly at first. "I'm so glad you're here," she said. "I've been waiting so long for this moment." She took a deep breath, her face softened and the light returned to her eyes. "It wasn't easy my little one but you made it… I made it… we made it together. And here we are, you and me." Then came the silence of the gaze, the moment of re-connection, the affirmation of the bond.

A month or so after the birth I was over at Heidi's place, drinking tea and watching mother and child playing with a rag ball on the kitchen carpet, - not mother playing with child but mother and child playing together. Over the years I've had countless opportunities to observe mothers interacting with their infants but the synchronicity between Heidi and Peter had me spellbound. When the game finished, it was by reciprocal agreement. Heidi picked up her son, sat down at the table and produced a substantial breast for their mutual satisfaction. "You seem to be getting along well together," I said. She looked up from her maternal connection. Her smile said everything.

CHAPTER FOUR

Merging Realities

Heidi's quest for a vaginal birth was an impressive display of personal determination. Stepping boldly out of character, this unassuming and generally compliant woman took it upon herself to challenge the experts and to get what she wanted. What makes her actions even more remarkable is that she could give no rational reason for her convictions. Her sense that something was missing from the birth of her daughters is hardly the kind of compelling evidence required to impress the medical establishment; yet six months after the birth of her son, she was even more convinced she had made the right choice. When asked about the reasons for her tenacity she would simply shrug her shoulders and say, "I just knew it was the right thing to do."

While this response might seem evasive there is good reason to believe that, based upon her own experience and understanding, Heidi was simply telling her truth. The chances are she was not responding to an idea created by her rational mind but to a thoughtless and wordless sense of knowing we call intuition or wisdom. As we all know, the human brain is an incredibly complex piece of biological engineering, and I am not about to expose my limited knowledge by attempting to offer a detailed neurological explanation for Heidi's intuitions and actions. Using the broadest of brushstrokes however, I would like to overview the basic structures and functions of the human brain to establish a framework for subsequent discussions.

The Fragmented Brain

Stated simply, it is generally accepted that our brain is made up of three major interconnected regions. At the center the brain-stem region contains the most basic structures, reflecting the earliest stages of our evolutionary journey into consciousness. This is the place of the instincts, the basic tools of survival, including the 'flight, freeze or fight' responses of the autonomic nervous system. Over time along with other mammals, we developed another layer that serves to regulate this primal reptilian brain and coordinate an increasingly differentiated range of internal experiences, from basic bodily functions to feelings and emotions. Identified as the limbic system, these circuits provide critical linkages between our internal world and our external environment. This is the stuff of the senses from which we experience our inherent sociability, including our ability to sense the internal states of others. Circumstantial and emotional memories, both individual and collective are encoded in this region and experienced not only through the brain, but also as a felt sense in the body. Herein lies our common relational heritage and information retrieved from this region is commonly referred to as intuition.

Limbic activity is penetrating and ubiquitous. Receiving and transmitting information, it reaches down into the brain-stem region and up into our most recent evolutionary resource, the mighty neo-cortex. This is where we step beyond the territory inhabited by other mammals and move into an abstract and symbolic world of our own creation. Five times larger than the other two regions combined, the neo-cortex is the home of the intellect providing us with our capacities for rational thought, language, reflection and creativity. This incredible neurological network makes it possible for us to step back from the immediacy of subjective experience, to create a symbolic world that can be modified and manipulated ad infinitum. In this world of abstract thoughts, we create and reflect upon the possibilities that enable us to comprehend, predict and control our environment. If our scientific and technological achievements seem impressive, consider the commonly held view that we are still using only a fraction of our neo-cortical capacities. With such potential the rational optimist might be excused for believing we have what it takes to solve any problem that comes along, from the threat of climate change to the shortage of Budweiser in Bellingham.

The trouble is that, left to its own devices, the neo-cortex can conjure up realities that resemble psychotic states, constrained only by the intellectual parameters of propositional logic and sustained through negotiated consensus – an agreement among those who are supposed to know. But it has no way of knowing who we really are and what serves our best interests. As the vehicle for our curiosity, it can never tell us what we need or what we should be curious about. Unless it is informed about these things, this wondrous piece of equipment is compelled to operate in a vacuum of superficial pragmatism, constantly struggling to solve the problems of its own making. Essentially, the neo-cortex facilitates our ability to think, but it is not the creator of our thoughts. In other words the evolutionary gift that offers our freedom can also lock us into a labyrinth of lunacy.

Nature did not design the neo-cortex to work in isolation: it is part of an interconnected complex system in which each cell and segment is set up to inform every other cell and segment. The deeper layers of this system – the reptilian and limbic regions – contain thoughtless memories and wordless realities that are essentially non-negotiable. Viewed from the current reality of the neo-cortex, information from these regions may be seen as primitive or inferior, but the blending of instinct and intuition is the foundation of our wisdom; the essential grounding for our insatiable curiosity. This is a place from which we know what we need, from the most basic elements of physical survival to the natural state of well being and our inherent relatedness to all·things. Only when intellect and wisdom are brought together can we begin to talk in terms of human intelligence.

So, if the human brain is designed to function in this elegant and integrated way, why are we in such a fragmented and disconnected mess? If we can navigate the space between the earth and the moon, what prevents us from exploring the space between one human being and another? If well being is a natural condition, why have we created so much discontent and despair in our pursuit of happiness? And if we are indeed connected to all things, why are we fighting each other to consume what's left of the planet's dwindling resources?

The blending of instinct and intuition is the foundation of our wisdom; the essential grounding for our insatiable curiosity ... Only when intellect and wisdom are brought together can we begin to talk in terms of human intelligence.

It's not that the intellect hasn't attempted to address such questions. In the western world there is no shortage of theories about our current evolutionary, genetic, biological and psychological condition. However, having framed the issues in these ways, the intellect is bound to seek solutions from its own perspective as a detached observer. Consequently the solutions it creates are limited to external forms of intervention – an impressive array of biological, psychological, sociological, political and ideological remedies that stretch further and further away from the understanding and subjective experience of the recipients. How many of us can honestly say we understand what the experts have to say about our bodies, our brains, our beliefs, our sexuality, our relationships, our societies, our cultures and the ecology of our planet? And if we don't understand, how can we possibly question their strategies?

Yet in her own way, Heidi did question the beliefs of the experts, and in so doing, she changed the course of life for herself, her son and consequently, for future generations. Her challenge was not based upon scientific discourse or even intellectual reason. All she did was suspend her disbelief and pay attention to the wordless voice on the inside. No matter what she had been taught to believe and what the experts had to say, she was compelled by a state of knowing that she refused to ignore. Such intuitive knowledge is generally dismissed by the rational mind and assigned to the category of mysticism, but it is no more mysterious than any other aspect of the human psyche. Despite the common western belief that intuition represents a lower form of knowledge than that generated by the intellect, this is a distinctively cultural perspective. Many renowned writers on this topic, most notably Ken Wilber, have continued to argue that when developed, intuition actually represents a heightened state of

How many of us can honestly say we understand what the experts have to say about our bodies, our brains, our beliefs, our sexuality, our relationships, our societies, our cultures and the ecology of our planet? And if we don't understand, how can we possibly question their strategies?

consciousness and the deepest level of knowing. In his book *Evolution's End*, Chilton Pearce suggests:

> *Intuition seems to fade around the age of seven if it is not developed, and developing it requires modeling and nurturing. The function fails to unfold either through lack of recognition and guidance, or through direct discouragement, as when parents consider such events to be pathological or psychotic. (p.150)*

Later he notes:

> *Without this intuition, we develop an intellect compulsively trying to compensate by engineering our environment and each other. This contributes to our living like 'armed crustaceans eternally on the alert' against a world we can't trust and curtails full development of our highest structures. (p.151)*

Could it be that our intellects are actually searching in all the wrong places for what we already know? I realize the seekers of enlightenment commonly advance this proposition, but it has also received impressive support from many celebrated men and women of western science including Albert Einstein. As Michael Polanyi documented in his 1958 book *Personal Knowledge* scientific breakthroughs most commonly occur when logic and reason are applied to an idea or insight that arises unexpectedly from a realm of knowing that is anything but scientific. In such moments of revelation the investigator ceases to be an observer and becomes an integral part of the phenomena under investigation. In other words, the answer becomes known before it is explicated and verified scientifically. In their initial presentation, such answers may appear to be illogical, irrational or paradoxical but once known, they have the power to change the course of scientific enquiry and reward the recipient with a Nobel Prize. Fifty years ago, the suggestion that science is the act of rationalizing what we already know would have seemed absurd, but with the recognition that human consciousness is an integral part of an interconnected universe, perhaps the time has come for us to liberate our intuition from the dark ages.

We may never understand how or why Heidi decided to reject the voices of authority, bracket off the messages of her rational mind and listen to the deeper voice. What I do know is that this new information gradually became assimilated

The human brain with all its complexity is not our master – it's our servant.

into her beliefs about herself and the world. I'm not suggesting she moved into some altered or transcendental state; on the contrary she remained a pillar of firmly grounded pragmatism. Yet some fundamental shift did take place. In a conversation with Judith some eighteen months after the birth of her son, she said:

> *You know my struggle wasn't so much with Dr. Quigley as with myself. Even in the birthing room, I was still telling myself that he was probably right and I was risking everything with my stubbornness. At one point I felt so guilty and helpless that I actually prayed for forgiveness. When I got home, I thanked God for making it all okay. The funny thing is that, in spite of all the doubts, this was probably the first time that I ever actually took charge of my life and made a really important decision on my own behalf. And, you know what? – I now know I made the right decision. I still can't explain why I did what I did; it was just a feeling. Perhaps we all know far more than we think, eh?"*

In my opinion this insight goes straight to the heart of the matter. The human brain with all its complexity is not our master – it's our servant. In taking charge of her life, Heidi responded to her intuition and despite resistance, she eventually convinced her rational mind to assimilate the

I am capable of thinking and acting on my own behalf, regardless of my genetic history, biological make-up, environmental influences and current circumstances.

unconventional wisdom. When this inner knowing is acknowledged and integrated, intellectual growth pursues a pathway that enables us to make intelligent decisions in our own best interests. If the intellect is cut off from these sources of information, its only internal option is to default to our most primitive survival impulses. The outcome is nothing less than a sophisticated form of psychopathy; capable of rationalizing the most inhuman and self-destructive acts in the name of righteousness. If you have any doubts about this look beneath the religious, cultural, ideological and sentimental regalia of the world we have created and invite your soul to report back.

The Intuitively Deprived Infant

The simple truth is that if we are cut off from our own intuition, we cannot nurture it in our children. If we are not prepared to take charge of our lives, we can hardly expect our kids to become self-responsible. So as always, it is we who must begin to do the work. To keep the rational mind engaged, I would like to set out with a simple working proposition: *I am capable of thinking and acting on my own behalf, regardless of my genetic history, biological make-up, environmental influences and current circumstances.* If this seems obvious or trite you should also be aware that such a statement is completely incompatible with the propositions that continue to direct the course of the biological, medical and psychological sciences. If you need to be convinced, you might like to try a few simple experiments. Lift up your arm and put it down again. Who made that decision? At your next meal, without permission or warning eat from someone else's plate. Was this action the product of my instruction, your own volition or did the Devil make you do it? If you are still unconvinced, devise more complex experiments, systematically recording the data until you have sufficient evidence to confirm that you are at the controls. If you choose to dismiss these suggestions on the grounds that they are all rather silly, I would agree with you wholeheartedly. My only point is that, without direction, even the most touted rational minds of science, theology and philosophy can be as inane and deceptive as they can be insightful and revealing.

My second proposition is drawn from what has already been discussed and, hopefully, warrants more serious attention: *In making decisions and acting on my own behalf, I have access to a vast body of learning and information that is not contained within, or presented through, the conscious mind.* In exploring this proposition you can consciously act upon your intuitions or 'gut feelings' and evaluate the outcomes. But if you wish to explore the full extent of this resource, you must temporarily suspend your dealings with the outside world and focus your attention on the inside experience. The key is to disengage the rational mind from its incessant search for 'understanding' and accept that the only goal is the experience itself. As my old therapist used to say, "get out of your head and come to your senses." In the absence of the intellect there are a number of activities, such as meditation and bodywork that can service your unfettered curiosity. The challenge is to train your conscious mind to sit back and listen to the silence. It is unlikely you will be suddenly rewarded with a rush of intuitive wisdom - these things

> *In making decisions and acting on my own behalf, I have access to a vast body of learning and information that is not contained within, or presented through, the conscious mind.*

The key is to disengage the rational mind from its incessant search for 'understanding' and accept that the only goal is the experience itself.

take time, commitment and patience.

In all of this the implications are that we all bring far more information into this world than we can ever accumulate during our brief residency on this planet. We know what has gone before and what we need to support our passage through life. From the moment of our conception this knowledge provides the foundation for all we subsequently learn about ourselves and each other on this mortal field trip. If we lose touch with this wisdom we abandon ourselves and are destined to seek meaning and purpose from the outside, creating an infinitely complex collage of illusionary approximations.

My dear friend and colleague Leanne Rose-Sladde, the mother of two delightful young boys once remarked that, unlike household appliances, children are not delivered with a manual and a life long warranty. A university professor with many years of experience working with children and youth, Leanne is a recognized authority on parenting practices. Yet in her own parenting, she frequently found herself questioning the theories she was obliged to teach and reacting negatively whenever her children failed to respond 'appropriately'. In one of our discussions she said:

"Eventually I came to realize that my kids are quite capable of letting me know what they need in their own way. Of course they've always been good at telling me what they want but that's a different matter. At first I found it easier to read Jared (age three) until I began to approach Daniel (age six) with the same curiosity. The neat thing is that the more I manage to understand their worlds, the more they seem able to understand mine. This alone helped me to put a lot of the old theories and techniques on the back burner. I guess you'd say we are all working and learning through our relationships."

What interests me most is that these two women, Heidi and Leanne arrived at a very similar place from very dissimilar points of departure. Perhaps children are delivered with a manual after all – a sort of universal *vade mecum* available to all and modified from one generation to the next. Like all mammals we know instinctively how to care for our young, but the evolution of human consciousness makes it possible for us to choose how to raise our children, with or without the collective wisdom of the manual. I'm not sure about the life long warranty, but I'm prepared to bet that children who are raised according to this manual will develop the resources to lead more self directed and fulfilled lives than those raised according to the prescriptions of the experts. Ideally these two sources of knowledge would be combined to make 'conscious parenting' the order of the day, but as things stand it's unlikely the authorities will ever be inclined to test out such a hypothesis.

The Infant in the Adult Mind

Most experts attempt to understand infants by watching them. Since babies are not able to talk about their inner experiences, these observers make inferences based upon their preferred theories of infancy and child development. Broadly speaking, their perspectives tend to be located on an established continuum of beliefs. At one end are those who view the infant as a biogenetic organism evolving in accordance with some pre-programmed developmental timetable. At the other we have those who see the infant as a passive creature waiting to be molded by environmental influences. Somewhere in the middle we find those who attempt to combine both perspectives in a variety of 'interactional' models. This continuum is of course, a reflection of the never-ending 'nature versus nurture' debate, and each point along the way is a complex formulation created and defended by a consensus of rational minds.

Then there are the clinicians who draw their conclusions from memories reported by their adult patients. While these folks are interested in the subjective experiences of childhood, the relationship between an infant experience and a recollection constructed by the adult mind many years later is to say the least, remote. These practitioners also rely upon their own particular theoretical perspectives in order to interpret and classify the presented and repressed memories of their clients. In this sense their observations are even further removed from the phenomena they seek to understand.

Having been a university student for nine years, I can attest to the fact that academics have amassed an impressive array of evidence to support, and occasionally challenge, their various stances. As a professional in the field, I have certainly drawn upon this body of information to guide my work with both children and adults. Once again, it's important to make a distinction between abstract knowledge based upon external observations and subjective knowing drawn from direct experience. This distinction is central to psychology as a whole, but it is particularly pertinent when it comes to understanding the experiential world of a pre-verbal child. Such understanding can only occur when both parties, adult and child, share the same experiential frame of reference.

The basic problem is that the observational stance assumed by the rational adult mind makes it impossible to comprehend the subjective world of the infant. The perspective of the observer is mediated by thoughts, symbols and language, while the infant's experience is direct and immediate. This is a world that can only be grasped through the senses, requiring a suspension of the brain's intellectual and imaginative faculties. The basis for understanding shifts from external observation to the creation of a lived-in experience that engages the fullness of the senses. Without this shift the observer is in the same position as a musicologist attempting to experience the magic of a Mozart symphony by notating and analyzing the score. Clearly, a full appreciation of Mozart's work requires a combination of both positions, but without the lived in sensual experience, its essence is lost.

In psychotherapy, this form of understanding is often referred to as 'accurate empathy' – the ability to respond to what the other is experiencing by placing oneself in the position of that person. From the perspective of the rational mind, this is a complex process in which the therapist responds to a multitude of visual, auditory, sensory and energetic cues presented by the client. At the intuitive level, it is also a natural ability made possible through the brain's limbic system. It has been widely noted for example, that newborn babies respond to each other empathetically, particularly in intensive care units where an infant is in pain or discomfort. Adults who wish to incorporate this level of empathy into their observations must train their minds to leave spaces for such information to be accessed and considered.

Our natural empathic potential is limited only by our ability to access our senses. This ability can be consciously enhanced through various cognitive, meditative and body awareness techniques; some therapists set out to train themselves in this way. Among adults empathy is often precipitated when one person reveals something about his or her inner world that arouses an associated feeling within the other. The result is a sense of knowing and connection that

Newborn babies respond to each other empathetically, particularly in intensive care units where an infant is in pain or discomfort.

transcends words and thoughts. Such expressions as "I can relate to that" do not do justice to what has actually taken place. Since the exchange is essentially energetic rather than cognitive, the word "resonance" is often used but even this term doesn't capture the substance of the subjective wordless experience.

To the rational mind, relating empathetically to pre-verbal children appears particularly difficult since they are not able disclose their inner experiences like thoughtful and reflective adults. Yet I would argue, the very opposite is the case. Because their worlds are uncluttered by the abstractions of the intellect, they invite us to go directly to that place of knowing where intuition and empathy are grounded. If you have questions about this, I suggest you go and hang out with a baby. If you can allow yourself to move with the infant's energy, responding rather than leading, you will find yourself being drawn back into the long lost world of your own infancy. This will not be in the form of mental images or memories, but as cerebral and bodily sensations. You might find this awkward at first but if you remain open to the experience, allowing the child to set the agenda, your adult thoughts and self-image will dissolve into the simple awareness of being in the moment with another human being. The baby's smiles and gurgles will arouse sensations of pleasure and feelings of joy, and you will find your body wanting to move in concert. His or her curiosity will invite you to look at the world again as if for the first time. If the infant becomes distressed, you will be led to your own place of discomfort. At this point you will probably be tempted to step back into your adult role in order to assuage the baby's discomfort and elicit some expression of contentment. Try to recognize this as your need and resist the temptation. The infant is in a constant state of learning and every sensation and emotion is an integral part of this process. The chances are, your desire to shape that process is more a reaction to your own experience and beliefs than a response to what the infant is seeking to learn. Unless there is some obvious need for adult intervention, your energetic and empathic presence is all that is required. The object of the exercise is to use your senses to understand, and the longer you

Their most primary concern is not the discomfort itself but the fear that they will be abandoned in this place.

stay there, the more natural it will become. When the episode is over and you return to your abstract world, you may think you have learned something about babies, but what you have really achieved is to re-learn something about yourself.

What you discover may well come as an insult to your intellect. Babies live in the 'eternal now' and invite us to join them in that timeless place of direct experience. Their learning is not abstract and sequential but immediate and holistic, and every moment contains an infinite storehouse of information. Here they are at one with themselves, seeking information from the outside and knowing what they want on the inside. They can lead and follow in responsive and reciprocal ways, and if we can participate without imposing our own interests, we will begin to re-learn what they already know. The more we allow them to have their own experience, the more we are able to understand and respond to their needs and expectations.

This does not mean babies need or expect to be comfortable and happy at all times. Their moments of discomfort are as essential to their learning as their moments of joy and contentment. What they expect at such times is connection and what they need is a mirror, provided by an empathic, loving and caring other, to assure them that their inner world is being recognized on the outside; that they are being seen and heard. Their most primary concern is not the discomfort itself but the fear that they will be abandoned in this place. The mirror confirms they are not alone and becomes the vehicle through which the infant Self can make its own way into the world.

I have already outlined the essential ingredients of empathic mirroring in the above discussion, but given its critical role in supporting the emergence of the Self, I will have much more to say on the topic as we move along. Meanwhile I'm not suggesting that we allow babies to remain cold, wet, hungry or physically distressed for experiential reasons. Clearly the time will come when adult intervention is desirable or necessary. My position is that the necessity and timing of such intervention will become immediately apparent to an adult who is empathetically and energetically attuned to the child. Such decisions are a response to the expectations and experience of the infant rather than to the wishes of the adult, or some predetermined strategy or schedule. We need to recognize that babies require a variety of experiences and allow them to control their own learning.

What Babies Expect

We also need to understand that babies do not see us as we see them. They do not observe or judge us; they experience us directly through their senses. Their learning is constant and immediate rather than reasoned and reflective. Their primary objective is experiential and not goal-directed in the linear sense. Unless their most basic physical needs are being denied, what they seek cannot be understood in terms of specific events or outcomes. From the moment of conception, their learning is guided by a set of expectations drawn from the collective experience of past generations, and by the time of their birth that state of expectancy is already augmented with information gleaned from their experience in the womb. This inherent ability to not only absorb but to organize this information may well form the core of what we think of as the Self.

From the outside, the most essential need is for contact – an affirmation of the connection to mother and through her, to life in general. At birth babies immediately look for a human face, expecting contact with the eyes of the mother they already know. If mother is not available, they will look elsewhere but attachment to a surrogate, often called 'imprinting', can never replace the bond already established with the mother.

It seems that somewhere within her strata of intuitive knowing, mother carries the same set of expectations. As Jean Liedloff has noted, if mother is not able to re-establish this bond immediately after the birth of her child, her experience will be one of grief – the loss of her baby – and her natural response will be to go into a state of mourning. If the baby is presented later, she cannot simply abandon her mourning and reassume mothering as though nothing had happened. The likelihood is that her feelings will turn to guilt and she will begin to display the symptoms of what we in the West call "postpartum depression." Is it possible that this common diagnosis has something to do with our culture and contemporary birthing practices? From Liedloff's perspective, what babies expect comes from a place that is no longer in harmony with the world we have created. If this is so then we need to ask ourselves whether this is a broken link in the evolutionary chain, or have we used our intellects to take us out of the natural order?

Liedloff's concept of the "continuum" is similar to what I referred to earlier as the "manual" - an inherent understanding of nature's design and an intuitive awareness of our connection to the whole. The continuum represents our collective knowing and contains its own built-in sequence of learning in which the infant absorbs information experientially, according to his or her current state of readiness. Over time, this instinctual learning will be slowly integrated into the child's emotional and intellectual development, blending wisdom with rational thought. In terms of my own thesis, this clearly suggests that an infant should be allowed to be at the centre of his or her own learning from the outset. Within the continuum, no attempt should be made to program the child according to some abstract theory of development. The role of the parent is to remain connected to the infant while providing a wide variety of learning opportunities.

This natural course of learning is made possible through benevolent contact - what Liedloff calls the "in-arms experience". In her anthropological work with the Yequana people of Venezuela, she noticed how mothers carried their babies with them through all their daily activities, attending to their needs without making 'mothering' a separate project. In this way, the baby's on going needs are met as they arise in the moment and the mother's everyday life remains intact. Attention is not given according to cultural beliefs about parenting or made contingent upon the infant meeting specific behavioural expectations. Whatever the baby does is simply accepted, and no attempt is made to divert or train the child in 'acceptable' ways. Liedloff was particularly impressed by how mothers seemed to know instinctively when their child needed their dedicated attention. When she asked how they knew when the infant needed to feed, eliminate or make contact, it was obvious they didn't even understand the question.

Contrary to her own western beliefs about parenting, Liedloff became convinced that this intuitive, non-judgmental approach to child rearing established the foundation for children to grow up with a profound sense of their own 'rightness'. From birth onwards they are engaged in the world of the adults, and with the minimum of fuss and protection, they are allowed to explore this world in their own time and in their own way. Yequana mothers do not fear for their children, but operate from an untutored belief that the child has the innate capacity to learn through direct experience. Fathers become increasingly involved as this learning begins to incorporate the fundamentals of the social and cultural expectations. By this time, the youngster is assured of his or her inherent 'rightness' and ability to respond to whatever circumstances might arise. In other words, Yequana children are encouraged to follow their own pathway toward establishing their own sense of worth and personal autonomy as a foundation for learning the ways of their parents. In Liedloff's words: "…

the object of the child's activities, after all, is the development of self reliance. To give either more or less assistance than he needs tends to defeat the purpose" (p.84). The underlying assumption is that children naturally seek connection and wish to become active players in the social order. Paradoxical as it may seem, my years of working with discontented, angry and 'deviant' children has led me to the very same conclusion.

Infants born into western cultures are generally considered to be helpless, empty, and willful creatures who must be taught as quickly and effectively as possible to conform to the conscious and unconscious expect- ations of the parents.

By contrast, infants born into western cultures are generally considered to be helpless, empty, and willful creatures who must be taught as quickly and effectively as possible to conform to the conscious and unconscious expectations of the parents. To this end, thoughtful parents are inclined to love them, protect them, amuse them and, when deemed necessary, correct, distract and even punish them. Parents who seek expert advice may choose from a wide range of child rearing strategies designed to bring about the desired outcomes. More often than not their intuitive senses are repressed, or overridden, with little or no concern for the subjective experience of their child. Over time the child learns to assume the same perspective by turning away from his or her inner world in order to focus on whatever is happening on the outside. Add to this the common practices of contingent rewards and conditional love, and we have a formula in which the child's inherent motivations become distorted, and his or her sense of Self becomes increasingly dependent upon the responses of the external world. Deprived of innate curiosity and purpose, the youngster strives to gain the attention of parents whose primary concern is to have a 'good' child. Competing with a multitude of parental distractions, including other siblings, is all part of the game and as the child's sense of 'rightness' becomes increasingly drawn to the outside, he or she is gradually eased out of the continuum.

Inner Space: The Lost Frontier

While I am convinced that parental intuition and dedication are the essential elements in supporting an infant's inherent sense of rightness, purpose and competence, it might be useful to engage the rational mind in taking a theoretical peek beneath the surface of these primary relationships. In order to do this I begin by borrowing from the work of early object relations theorists, specifically D. W. Winnicot. This is a complex perspective that incorporates philosophical, psychological and clinical ideas and once again, I run the risk of oversimplification. Concerned primarily with the early development of the psyche, object relations represent the only enduring attempt to understand the infant's subjective experience, albeit from a predominantly psychoanalytic perspective.

I have already discussed how the unborn child is assumed to marinate in the womb, experiencing a state of symbiotic oneness with the mother. The first fleeting energetic separation occurs in that inevitable moment when she fails to respond in unison, leaving the unborn child suddenly isolated and alone. This, I suggest, is a highly charged somatic experience that creates our first confrontation with the Nemo, laying the foundation for the universal fear of abandonment. Winnicot and his colleagues did not address this primal event since their concern was with the later development of the human psyche, and their ideas were formulated well before the emergence of pre- and perinatal and somatic psychology as recognized disciplines. Through the lens of object relations, healthy separation from the mother is seen to occur as the child becomes progressively able to distinguish between inner reality and the external world - between the 'me' and the 'not-me'. In the period immediately following birth the infant makes no such distinction, regarding mother and her life-nurturing breast as aspects of the 'me'. Beginning with various forms of self-stimulation, the infant gradually shifts to exploring the physical world having learned how to use thumb and fingers to grasp and manipulate external objects. Almost invariably, these objects are checked out through the child's most beloved sensor – the mouth.

While these early exploratory behaviors may be seen as an attempt to close the gap between the external and internal worlds, the child becomes increasingly aware of another reality – one that exists beyond immediate experience. In this widening schism between the two realities, the child begins to lose the comforting illusion of subjective omnipotence – the sense that the objects of desire are the product of his or her own wishes. Winnicot and his colleagues coined the term "transitional space" to describe the expanding territory between the child and external world, most specifically the mother object. It is reasonable to assume that the anxiety created by this growing sense of separation may trigger the body 'memory' of mother's temporary absences during the pregnancy. In order to assuage this anxiety, the child will normally attach himself or herself to particular objects, claiming them as part of the 'me'. In many cases this need to maintain some sense of security in the unresponsive void will become focused on one particular possession - a representation of the missing mother that can be controlled and manipulated at will. The most common objects include blankets and stuffed toys, but the same service can be provided through familiar tunes, visual images and auditory sequences.

Teddy and the Blanket

These possessions referred to by Winnicot as "transitional objects", play a critical role in the developmental drama. Beyond their capacity to soothe and provide a substitute for the mother, they facilitate the first steps toward separation and independence by providing the infant with opportunities to satisfy his or her own needs and move beyond the expectation that mother will always be ready and available. With the development of cognition, transitional objects become symbols in the emerging psyche and over time, the child is able to 'keep them in mind' in dealing with mother's absence by constructing an image, or fantasy, about her. This provides the assurance of mother's existence, even when she is not physically present, and represents a pivotal stage in establishing the distinction between the 'me' and the 'not me'.

At the deepest level, transitional objects play an important role in laying the early foundations for subsequent self-definitions and personal autonomy. To this end, parents need to recognize the significance of the favored 'not-me' possession and allow the child full ownership and control over the object's treatment and destiny. I have often come across parents who became disturbed by their child's treatment of these objects, particularly where the parents had some understanding that the item in question may represent some form of 'mother' substitute. Anger and frustration directed toward the object were deemed to be offensive, or even pathological, and the associated behaviors were discouraged or sanctioned. In some cases, the parents chose to dispossess the child of the abused object, or make its availability contingent upon more desirable behavior. Apart from having to deal with the infant's subsequent distress, their actions removed a critical ingredient from the developmental recipe of the Self - the opportunity to challenge the arbitrary expectations and demands of the external world.

Within the natural course of development, transitional objects gradually lose their significance and symbolic meanings. The more children are encouraged to explore the territory between inner experience and external reality, the greater their sense of security and the less dependent they become on their attachment to specific objects. In effect they are learning to live in a relational world. As they develop cognitively, transitional space becomes progressively diverse, and the need-based fantasies are transformed into inventions of imagination that are no longer bound by the parameters of external reality. This is the arena of creativity from which artistic, interpersonal and spiritual expression will eventually emerge. As in the case of transitional objects, it is important for parents to understand that these imaginative excursions have their own inherent validity and no attempt should be made to challenge them, repress them, or bring them into line with the 'real' world.

Again I have worked with many parents who became concerned that their young son or daughter was straying too far from 'reality' and needed to be assured that this is not only normal, but also an essential aspect of psychic development. The ability to differentiate between inner and outer experience is an inherent aspect of the learning process and most children have everything they need to proceed at their own pace in their own time.

Throughout this period, parents need to be gentle and curious while making sure the external world remains accepting, interesting and accessible. Free from the fear of judgments and sanctions, children will openly share their inner experiences, not simply for approval, but more significantly, for affirmation of their internal reality; and this is where the availability of a reliable mirror is particularly important. The development of imagination is enhanced when they have access to a broad range of visual, auditory and sensual experiences. People, objects, pictures, sounds, emotions and social events are all grist for the mill, but the essential ingredient is that children should be free to create their own fantasies around whatever they choose.

> *Children should be free to create their own fantasies around whatever they choose.*

In western cultures parents often attempt to capture the child's inner life by imposing fantasies they consider normal and acceptable. But the child is not the creator of Mickey Mouse, or The Friendly Giant, and such impositions are more than likely to retard the development of the imagination and replace it with a life-long desire to be 'entertained.' In this way the child slips from being an active participant in life to a passive responder. I am convinced that this is why so many of us in North America have become addicted to external forms of stimulation and amusement.

The seeds of this dependency are sown when addicted adults feel the need to keep babies happy. As the youngster becomes increasingly demanding and the adults begin to tire, more gadgets and gimmicks are introduced until the day finally comes when television and video games take over. From that point on the child is well on the way to becoming a consumer of commercial fantasies. Effectively, the space between inner and outer reality is short-circuited and the primitive demands for pleasure and gratification are projected onto the external world. However hard they might try, parents who attempt to keep their entitled kids happy are fighting a losing battle, behaviorally, emotionally and, to their dismay, financially. From this beginning, the really smart kids will grow up as dedicated opportunists, scrambling to consume what's left of the earth's resources in a futile attempt to replace what they have lost. The majority, the losers, will sink into an apathetic learned helplessness to become the fodder for the aspirations of the elite. This is not intended to be a prediction of what might be, but a statement of the way things are.

There are many reasons why a boy or girl may choose to reject external reality, but as long as we have little interest in the subjective world of children, we will never understand.

In some cases, a child may choose to reject the objective world in favor of a reality that is inaccessible to outsiders. The term 'autism' is commonly used to identify this condition and it is generally attributed to some form of brain dysfunction that still confounds the experts. Like most psychobiological labels, the term explains absolutely nothing and offers no solution, other than the senseless prescriptions we call 'education' and 'treatment'. In my experience there are many reasons why a boy or girl may choose to reject external reality, but as long as we have little interest in the subjective world of children, we will never understand. Our tendency to objectify the child with a label and seek medical solutions demonstrates our own lack of imagination and our dependency upon the external world. In other words, we are reacting to our own deficiencies in exploring and managing transitional space. Again the question is whether or not an adult can do anything to rectify this learning deficiency and again, my answer is in the affirmative.

If I was to suggest you allow yourself to explore, even express your fantasies and learn how to distinguish them from the reality of everyday life, you may question my motives. You may assume I'm inviting you to sever your attachment to the objective and moral order, or promoting some half-baked form of therapy. This is not the case. I'm convinced we are all capable of stepping back into the 'continuum' without sacrificing our morality or threatening the security of our place in the world. All it takes is practice but in order to do this, you may feel safer with the support of a competent therapist. In this case, my only advice would be to choose very carefully.

Good Mommy, Bad Mommy

Before leaving the ubiquitous world of transitional space, I want to go back to the time when the child is assumed to live 'as one' with the mother, making no distinction between inner and outer reality. This is a non-verbal world of direct experience, in which the infant responds to immediate sensations of satisfaction and pleasure on the one hand, and discomfort and pain on the other. In the earliest phases of individuation, this dichotomized version of reality is projected onto the outside world where contact with any given object may be either positive or negative in any given moment. Since these are two distinct sensations, the child experiences them as stemming from two different objects. In the early stages, this applies as much to mother as to any other 'object', but here the developmental implications are particularly profound. Incorporating the mother into his or her own experience, any attribution to her is also applied to the child's own emerging sense of Self. In other words, the child internalizes the equation, "good Mommy" = "good me" and "bad Mommy" = "bad me." These early messages provide the generalized foundation for the subsequent development of what we call 'self-esteem' and may help to explain why children who are neglected or abused in infancy grow up with enduring questions about their own inherent worthiness.

Where nature is allowed to take its course, the dichotomized world of the infant becomes progressively differentiated with the development of perceptual and cognitive abilities. External objects become perceived as 'not me', and their qualities are recognized beyond their immediate impact. The simple 'good or bad' attributions of early infancy are gradually replaced by more complex mental constructs that enable the child to consider an increasing range of characteristics and potentials in every object and event. In particular the child comes to see Self and Other as separate, unique and complex beings. This is an essential step toward the creation of relationships in which the person is able to recognize, care about, and love another in his or her own right. The transformational aspect of this development is that 'good' mommy and 'bad' mommy are gradually incorporated into the same object – "the good mommy who just fed me is the same mommy who just left me, and even when she is not here, she continues to exist and will return." As the internalized image of mother becomes more separate, consistent, reliable and trustworthy, the child is able to tolerate her absences and find ways to manage these periods of aloneness. This is the groundwork for constructing subsequent relationships based upon trust, self-reliance and personal autonomy – the foundations of intimacy and love. The eminent child psychologist, Jean Piaget, coined the term 'object constancy' to describe this primary developmental task. If this natural process is interrupted in some way, the developmental implications can be far-reaching. For example a child's inability to attain object constancy is often a consequence of the 'good-bad' dichotomy being imposed upon the infant in response to his or her behavior. This occurs when parents or caretakers have failed to accomplish this developmental task for themselves and, through their black and white world-view, unwittingly pass their deficit on to their children.

At the broadest level, children who are unable to achieve a functional level of object constancy and separate effectively from the mother-object are destined to spend much of their adult lives searching for a 'good' replacement. The chances are their closest relationships will become enmeshed, while their thwarted need for individuation will continue to generate an effusive undercurrent of dissatisfaction and resentment – usually directed toward the unfortunate other. Having little sense of themselves as separate and integrated beings, they attach to others as objects of their own desires and gratification. In their inflexible psyche, they carry the image of the 'ideal' partner-object, but they will always be left wanting. Incapable of 'knowing' another, they 'fall in love' at the drop of a hat, but the cherished love-object will always fail and end up as a tarnished illusion. What they really fall in love with is the missing 'good me' and what they reject is the unacceptable or 'bad me' – but try telling them that!

Children who are unable to achieve a functional level of object constancy and separate effectively from the mother-object are destined to spend much of their adult lives searching for a 'good' replacement.

In case you're wondering about my own level of object constancy, I am not suggesting there are two kinds of people hanging around out there – developmentally arrested 'cling-ons' and fully individuated beings like you and me. The course of our personal development is a continuum that stretches across the entire life span, and individual differences must always be considered as a matter of degree. Personally I believe separating from our parents, particularly mother, is an on going task that none of us will ever fully complete. My concern here is with those interruptions of early childhood that, if left unresolved will continue to sabotage the overall development of Self and the creation of lasting and meaningful relationships. Such interruptions usually manifest themselves through recurring patterns of self-defeating behavior. Therapists, particularly those who work with couples, may choose to diagnose and address these problems in many different ways, but very few are prepared to dig this deeply into the pot. Who could blame them? As in medicine, the symptoms are so much more accessible and 'treatable' than the causes.

Separating from our parents, particularly mother, is an on going task that none of us will ever fully complete.

Returning to the matter of object constancy, children who have difficulty moving through this developmental task are likely to organize their subsequent thinking around rigid 'good' or 'bad', black or white, constructs. Once established, this simplistic mind-set is imposed on their perceptions and beliefs about themselves, others, and the world in general. Unable to tolerate ambiguity, their inherent curiosity is diminished and the neo-cortex is pressed into the service of 'forcing the data' into these two polarized categories.

The implications for cognitive development are obvious, but the impact on the evolution of Self, and the formation of relationships, is even more far-reaching. In their search for acceptance and rightness, children will naturally cling to the good attributions and present these qualities to the world in order to gain recognition and approval. Defined by Winnicott as the "false Self," this early attempt to control the impressions of others becomes a patterned way of surviving in an idealized, though potentially rejecting, world. Meanwhile, the 'bad' stuff is conveniently tucked away, hidden from the external world and effectively removed from consciousness. The container of this repressed material has been likened to a backpack that is carried into adulthood and, in many ways, resembles what Carl Jung referred to as the "Shadow." In the early formation of the psyche, these aspects of the rejected Self are transformed into fantasies and projected onto the external world whenever the conscious mind is off its guard, particularly during sleep. Here we find the demons under the bed and the monsters in the closet. In our culture these scary images are considered to be a normal part of growing up and we do our best to assure children that such ogres don't exist. Well they do, and the most effective way to support children through their quest for object constancy would be to invite them to get to know the demons and even befriend them. Before we sanitized them and created ridiculous animations, the original fairy tales served this very purpose. Strange as it may seem, you might be surprised at the ability and willingness of young children to explore whatever lies within them.

Once inside the head of an adult however, the monsters become securely locked into the closet of the unconscious, restrained by denial, shackled by inflexible beliefs and walled up behind compulsive behaviors. Unable, or unwilling, to appreciate the subtle and diverse qualities contained within any object, concept or event, the custodians cling to their rules, rituals, religions and righteousness. Projected by the unconscious onto the external world, the sources of evil can be attacked and destroyed without compunction or conscience. It's tempting to launch into a rant about the prevalence of such pathological fundamentalism in the modern world, but assuming you are equally concerned, I will spare you the burden of my catharsis. My primary point is that if this condition is indeed a reflection of our global development, there is no new ideology or cause that will rectify the deficit and save us from the consequences of our voluntary retardation. I use the word 'voluntary' on the understanding that most of us have what it takes to identify and resolve our basic developmental limitations and create new opportunities for our children. Until we do this however, we will continue to put our faith in leaders who are developmentally arrested - men and women who have no doubts about what's good and what's evil and have no hesitation in packaging the former and declaring war on the latter.

The Conscious Parent

If you think I'm asking far too much, you may be right. Please understand I have no illusions about some sudden and miraculous transformation in global consciousness – although, given what we know about developmental processes, such a quantum leap may not be beyond the realm of possibility. In his classic work *The Origin of Consciousness in the Breakdown of the Bicameral Mind*, Julian Jaynes describes how throughout history, human consciousness has moved through periods of rapid acceleration, much like the leaps that occur during early childhood. Despite my weary skepticism I still find some comfort when my aging 'New Age' friends and colleagues continue to tell me that we are now in throes of such a transformation. More 'realistically' however, what I am really wishing for is some recognition of the problem and a conscious shift in direction that can only be achieved one person at a time. Strategies for the dissemination of accurate information, combined with remedial and educational opportunities would certainly help to support the cause, but even in the most democratic societies, initiatives for change will only become effective through the will of an electorate that is already conscious and aware of its developmental condition.

Uncommitted or neglectful parents would have no interest in hearing the message, let alone be concerned about their parenting practices.

By the same token, I'm not scanning the horizon for the arrival of a new breed of parents – enlightened caregivers and teachers who will reverse the flow of mindless parenting and education by pointing our kids toward personal awareness and self-responsibility. Based upon Fritz Perls's cited belief that 'nothing can be changed until it's seen for what it is,' my modest ambition has been to invite adults who are concerned about the well being of children to examine our current parenting and educational practices and consider the options. I have taken this message out to whoever seemed inclined to listen through my client work, parent-training programs, conferences, newspaper articles, radio and television presentations and publications like this one.

All too often, parents who accepted the challenge have ended up expressing guilt or remorse about their parenting 'failures,' depreciating themselves in the process. To them, there are four points I would like to make.

- Uncommitted or neglectful parents would have no interest in hearing the message, let alone be concerned about their parenting practices.

- All concerned parents do the very best they can, given what they know and have received from their own parents.

- Whatever they consider to be their parenting deficiencies, their children have all the inner resources they need to move on and create the lives they want.

- Any child whose immediate needs are identified and addressed by the 'perfect parent' will be developmentally incapacitated. Allow me to explain.

An infant Self certainly needs love, nurturing and support to step forward in the world. Children need to be seen and heard for who they really are by those they know and trust. But the Self is not simply a passive receiver – its mission is to be an active player in a less than perfect world. Beginning with the struggle of birth, the emerging Self needs to know it can deal with adversity and take charge of its own destiny. Through these challenges, it develops its resilience, strength and tenacity.

> *The emerging Self needs to know it can deal with adversity and take charge of its own destiny.*

When parents or caretakers are not able or available to meet the child's immediate needs, a critical internal learning potential is triggered – the ability to call upon internal resources to ensure survival, continuity and well being. In this way, the child learns to develop an internal sense of security that is not dependent upon the ever-changing conditions of the external world.

The Good Enough Parent

The acclaimed Austrian psychologist Bruno Bettleheim created the notion of "good enough parenting" to describe how children are not only able to tolerate, but actually benefit from sporadic lapses in parental attention and attunement. In recent years, others have used this same term to identify parenting practices they regard as marginally adequate, but this is not what Bettleheim had in mind. The overall responsibility of the parent is to offer a loving, nurturing and consistent presence, not to provide some ideal response to every behavior or demand. Even if this were possible, such parenting would allow no freedom for the child to take charge of his or her own life. Parental absences and failures to respond are like mini encounters with the Nemo. Through these experiences, the emerging Self learns to draw from its own resources, while the ever-expanding mind is challenged to explore its inherent imaginative and creative potentials. Similarly in the critical area of mirroring, a 'perfect' parent who is able to accurately reflect every facet of a child's inner experience would leave nothing for that child to contribute on his or her own behalf. The missing or misread responses are the opportunities the child needs to bring forward the unseen aspects of the Self and negotiate their rightful place in the world. The child who is able to say to the world "that may be what you see, but this is who I really am" is on the pathway to self-realization. Unfortunately such children are few and far between. To this end, 'good enough' parents are actually 'ideal' parents and, paradoxical as it

> *The overall responsibility of the parent is to offer a loving, nurturing and consistent presence, not to provide some ideal response to every behavior or demand.*

might seem, their perceived imperfections are as essential to their child's development as all the thoughtful and intuitive attention they give to 'conscious' parenting.

Problems arise when one side of the equation is either overloaded or missing. The 'programmed' child who receives constant parental attention and concern will likely end up feeling invaded and helpless, while the overly neglected child will continue to struggle with a debilitating sense of abandonment. When I explain this principle to parents, they often ask how they might balance this equation effectively. While I always admire their dedication to the cause, such a question would make no sense to parents raised in Liedloff's 'continuum'. Of course I keep this observation to myself and begin by pointing out how babies learn to stand up by falling down. Acknowledging them as caring and committed parents, I try to assure them that, given the opportunity, children raised in a nurturing, loving and stimulating environment will take increasing levels of responsibility for their own learning. From birth onwards, their capacity to pursue their own course of curiosity and manage their own moments of displeasure and discomfort, is constantly expanding, along with their ability to ring the alarm when help is needed.

The experience of being alone is the fallow field in which the seeds of imagination, creativity and self-reliance are nurtured and ripened.

In providing this level of responsive freedom, parents must be able to separate their own needs and fears from those of the child. This is easier said than done, since parental over-indulgence and over-protection generally stem from the parent's own childhood deficits and fears. Without awareness these interruptions are imposed upon the youngster, breaking through delicate energetic boundaries and disturbing the natural flow of empathic energetic attunement between parent and child. Alternatively, when boundaries are respected and both parties are attuned, the child has the freedom to grow and the parents have the freedom to carry on with their own lives. This is not a parenting strategy; it is a mutually negotiated arrangement through which the child learns to manage transitional space by establishing a progressively autonomous place for the Self in relationship with others. In this, the experience of being alone is the fallow field in which the seeds of imagination, creativity and self-reliance are nurtured and ripened. 'Good enough' parents create the conditions in which this new unfolding life gains strength and confidence, from the inside out. In this way, they pave the way for both separation and connection.

To understand how this happens, it's important to remember that pre-verbal infants do not learn like adults. Their learning is multi-modal, engaging all the senses and the information they use is derived from a diverse range of sources. Unless they are traumatic or persistent, single events have relatively little impact on the whole. Learning is not limited to the neo-cortex. In responding to the developmental needs of the Self, the infant employs the senses experientially, connecting to the limbic system and the more primitive brain stem region. The messages received and assimilated are general and sensual, rather than specific and sequential. If this natural learning process is interrupted or overridden by external programming, the core ingredients of the Self will become isolated and disconnected from the whole. The knowing, accessible through authentic feelings and intuition, will be overpowered by the information that flows from the external world. In this way, the infant may become an obedient child, and eventually, a good student, but he or she will always be a diminished and disconnected human being, constantly searching for the missing piece.

In the theatre of the mind, adults and pre-verbal infants perform in very different realities. It would be presumptuous to conclude that the experiential world of the child is any less 'real' than the cognitively constructed world of the adult – in fact, many would argue that it is more authentic. In ideal circumstances these two spheres overlap to create a shared area of transitional space in which both parties are free to explore and negotiate together. Expressed through adult concepts and words, this might sound abstract and lofty, but if you spend time messing about with infants and toddlers as full and equal participants, the chances are you will find the boundaries of your thoughtful world being delightfully dissolved. When their reality is recognized and affirmed from the outside, children will gradually blend the two spheres into an integrated whole – an amalgam of direct experience and abstract thought. In childhood this provides the foundation for creative and expressive play. Taken into adulthood, people who are able to develop their intellectual potential, without losing contact with the sensual world of direct experience, never lose their ability, or their desire, to become engaged in spontaneous, non-competitive play. Whatever the constructed world might look like, they remain grounded in their senses, looking for the truth within themselves rather than relying upon the consensual validation of like minds. Their learning employs all the senses and when they act, they do so on their own behalf and not according to some social or moral prescription.

Caretakers who are cut off from the experiential world can offer only half the mirror, wittingly or unwittingly drawing the child away from the internal experience of the Self.

The ability, or inability, to integrate these two spheres of reality becomes particularly apparent in pre-school children. At this point, cognitive development is moving ahead by leaps and bounds, driven by the youngster's innate curiosity and natural desire to participate in the adult world. Caretakers who remain connected to their own direct experience are able to stay attuned to the child, affirming one reality while opening the doors to the other. On the other hand, caretakers who are cut off from the experiential world can offer only half the mirror, wittingly or unwittingly drawing the child away from the internal experience of the Self. This is not a time for prescriptive parenting or teaching. I am talking here about an interactive process in which adults and children engage their senses and imaginations to 'play' between two domains, each taking a turn in leading the other in a game of mutual learning and understanding. The delicate task of the adult is not to direct this process but to establish the conditions through which this can occur naturally. Allow me to offer an example.

The Meeting Place

At a time when I was feeling particularly burdened by my professional responsibilities, Judith suggested I might like to refresh my spirit by spending a morning with a group of twenty pre-schoolers involved in an experimental learning program. Given my schedule it was a ridiculous idea but two days later I entered an old portable building in the middle of nowhere and disappeared for six hours.

Like a stranger at a cocktail party I stood in the doorway of the 'Adventure Room,' considering how I might insinuate myself into the action without drawing too much attention. As expected, the place was full of little kids, some clumped around tables, others wandering from group to group like shoppers at a Saturday market. But this was no socialized ritual, and the free-floating energy was sufficient to offend the senses of anyone who believed children should play quietly.

I couldn't make out what was holding the attention of each group, but it would have been presumptuous of me to step into the role of a wanderer and find out. I also wanted to avoid being intrusive - not wishing to impose an adult presence on the proceedings. Or so I thought. Meanwhile, beneath all this rationalization, my belly was trying to tell me the truth: and the truth is that I am shy, and have been for as long as I can remember. As a child, I covered my inhibitions with awkward pretenses; always scared I would be found out. In early adulthood, I learned how to hide behind roles and social competencies. As a schoolteacher, my secret was always quietly contained beneath the assigned mantle of authority and later, as a psychotherapist with 'Dr.' attached to my name, I could always seek safety in status and label if necessary. Yet there I was once again, a bashful little boy with a hole in his belly standing in a doorway asking the same old questions and fearing rejection.

True to form, my brain came to the rescue and I headed for a chair in the corner where I could safely settle down and take it all in through my psychologists' eye. But my arrival had already been noticed. Gail Goldsmith, the program leader, rose from one of the mystery groups, waved a welcoming hand in my direction, and with a smile that could have dissolved the doubts of any tremulous child, strolled over to a piano by the window. Still standing, she tinkled out a few notes and began to sing:

> "Here comes Gerry ... Gerry, Gerry Gerry.
> He's come to play with us today,
> Let's say hello to Gerry."

The noise level dropped considerably and while the overall flow of energy in the room didn't seem to be unduly affected by the interruption, I was left in no doubt about being the focus of attention – at least momentarily. As the adult prepared his speech and the little boy prepared for the worst, Gail Goldsmith made both redundant by gliding over to offer her own personal greeting. "Welcome to Wonderland," she said. "Please have fun – Judith tells me you could use some." Then with a smile and a touch on the hand, she returned to her group at the table. This fleeting introduction was the only permission I needed to become a *bonae fide* wanderer. In the most elegant way, this young woman had acknowledged the hesitant adult and assured the doubtful child of his freedom. So with our inhibitions 'tucked away for another day,' we stepped boldly into that oddly familiar place.

I would love to share with you all that I experienced and learned on that day, but the memories and words of a settled and reflective mind could never re-capture the essence of what actually took place. With no goals to accomplish or expectations to meet, I found myself completely caught up in the mundane and fascinated by the obvious. As my imagination gleefully pushed beyond the boundaries of rationality, I put aside all sense of context.

My relationships with the other kids were not constrained by particular friendships or allegiances. Riding my own curiosity and excitement, I moved from one adventure to the next, relishing the freedom to choose without permission or consultation. Eventually I settled into a group that was creating a collage from an assortment of pictures scattered about the table. Lisa, a very serious little girl with tightly woven pigtails, explained that they were taking turns to add a picture, which David conveniently demonstrated by placing a photograph of sailboat next to a painting of an eagle before announcing, "We're all going on holiday." Everybody cheered. When Robbie invited me to take a turn, I chose a drawing of a little boy holding onto a red balloon and slid it between a ballerina and a chimpanzee. "What's the story?" asked Lisa, "we have to keep the story going." "Well, we can do anything we want on our holiday," I answered without thinking. "Oh yeah," said Rachel, reaching for a gaudy hamburger poster. David rubbed his tummy and we all laughed.

It wasn't all laughter and delight. Throughout the day, the unfinished business of my own childhood constantly interrupted the flow - moments of jealousy or frustration when I felt the old urge to withdraw, sulk or hit out in anger. The feelings were real, although I always knew my adult Self was carefully monitoring, ready to step in should things get out of hand. For the others, there was the ubiquitous Gail Goldsmith who always seemed to appear at precisely the right time – not only to mediate disputes and assuage hurts, but also to rekindle curiosity and integrate learning. As a child, I had no particular interest in how she was able to do this - it just happened. Later when I returned to adulthood however, I was determined to discover her secret and with her support, arranged for a film crew to move in the following week. The result was a movie we called "The Teachable Moment," and I'm delighted to say it went on to take first prize as "Best Documentary" at the Alberta Film and Television Awards.

Having watched this movie many times over, I continue to be amazed by the natural blend of attunement, intuition and gentle mirroring Gail Goldsmith brought into her encounter with each child. It was her ability to stay in touch with the group as a whole that tugged at my curiosity. Whenever I asked her about this she struggled to come up with an answer. In one conversation she said, "Until you started asking questions, I'd never really thought about these things. It's not that I spend my time watching the children; I'm always far too busy for that. I'm not even listening to what's going on around me – not consciously anyway." With this revelation, it occurred to me that this graceful young woman was probably using the same abilities found in all effective parents and teachers. We have all heard stories of mothers who just 'know' when their child is on the way home or is in some kind of trouble, and while we may not understand how this actually happens, such experiences are relatively commonplace. Thinking back to my days as a classroom teacher I now realize I also had the ability to dedicate my attention to one student while being aware of the class a whole. What made Gail Goldsmith remarkable was not that she possessed unique qualities but the degree to which these natural faculties were developed and refined.

In our personal contacts, what impressed me most about Gail was the intensity of her presence. Whenever we were together, I just knew she was fully 'there' and I was the central focus of her concern - as both a child and an adult. Among the children she moved seamlessly from one reality and another without tension or pretension. Unlike many members of her profession, she didn't walk around dishing out approval and disapproval in an attempt to choreograph the learning. We were not a group of kids walking that fine line between our innate curiosity and the imposition of adult judgments and expectations. Her very presence was sufficient to legitimize whatever was being learned with an assurance of 'rightness' for each child – me included. Yet it was clear to us all that she was the adult in the group, and she brought this sense of calm security into every encounter. Sometimes she would enhance our discoveries by introducing new possibilities, but always through gentle invitations rather than expectations or demands. There was nothing condescending in her attitude. Her enthusiasm for every revelation was infectious and confirmed that whatever was being learned was of value to us all. My adult mind continued to ponder on how she accomplished all this but as we left the old portable building after that very special day, she offered a priceless clue. Walking across the parking lot, I took her arm and said, "Thank you again Gail; that was absolutely wonderful." To which she smiled and replied, "Yes, aren't they?"

After listening to my enthusiastic account of my experience one of my colleagues summed it up as "an interesting exercise in regression" – an episodic return to a former period of development. I disagreed wholeheartedly. To me she was

> *It really is possible for adults to share transitional space with children by consciously stepping outside their familiar boundaries of reality.*

simply reiterating the traditional linear view that each stage of development is rendered obsolete by the one that follows. In my mind this was not a mindless lapse into the past, but a fully conscious, lived-in experience of the present. This was a reality existing side by side with the world constructed through my intellect. In this place my learning was grounded in immediate feelings, sensations and transitory thoughts with little concern for the accumulation of knowledge for future considerations. Yet at no point did I abandon my adult integrity. At some level I always knew I would never really lose myself in the experience. Throughout it all the seasoned Self of Gerry Fewster remained as a rational and vigilant figure in the background, like a researcher who temporarily suspends experimental operations to re-examine the raw data. How needed and timely it was.

Only later when my emotions began to settle, did I try to make sense of it all. Given time for reflection my rational mind began to do what it does best, artfully blending subjectivity with objectivity to create workable propositions. In this case I concluded that it really is possible for adults to share transitional space with children by consciously stepping outside their familiar boundaries of reality – in much the same way as we suspend disbelief when we become immersed in a play or a movie. This is not an abandonment of rationality; it actually involves a conscious decision to redefine the context - what social psychologists refer to as a 're-definition of situation.' My choice was to redefine the old portable as a 'meeting place' and to invest myself as a fully committed and curious participant.

By placing my adult agenda on hold I opened myself up to a full spectrum of learning, from the raw sensations in the body to the refined reflections of the intellect – the life-affirming reconnection of the 'knower' with the 'knowledge.' What I actually learned or relearned, was fascinating stuff, but the questions that most occupied my mind were about how and why I did what I did, without being guided by coherent thoughts and conscious intentions. After much deliberation I came to the conclusion that I was acutely aware of what was taking place within and around me, and my aspirations remained specific and focused. In other words my learning was both organized and purposeful. In those few hours I made countless choices on my own behalf, even though I would have been hard pressed to specify the reason. In this sense it was business as usual. I was simply doing what I've always done; attend to my transitory interests while seeking a place for my Self in the scheme of things. The only difference was that I had given my overworked intellect a few hours off. Even without the assistance of this most loyal servant, there I was exploring my potentials and carving out my own niche in my own way.

By placing my adult agenda on hold I opened myself up to a full spectrum of learning, from the raw sensations in the body to the refined reflections of the intellect.

From this I conclude that we are who we are, whatever our circumstances and wherever we happen to be on the developmental continuum. Once again I am affirming my belief that the Self is not a product of our individual experience but the central motivational force in our lives. Psycho-biological processes and imperatives may have their place, but the need of the Self to be recognized, elaborated and expressed lies at the very core of our emotional, cognitive, relational and even physical development; from conception onwards it is the internal reference that both directs and organizes our learning. Its primary concern is not with who we want to be, but who we really are, and its essential learning context is the human relationship.

The need of the Self to be recognized, elaborated and expressed lies at the very core of our emotional, cognitive, relational and even physical development; from conception onwards it is the internal reference that both directs and organizes our learning.

My purpose in telling this story is to illustrate how, in the optimum state, the cerebral world of the adult and the more direct world of the infant are actually interwoven aspects of the same experience. Both are equally real and essential for the development of Self, although each requires its own distinctive style of accessing and assimilating information. Simply stated, infants learn by employing all of the senses and rely upon internal experience for affirmation. Adults, on the other hand, are inclined to construct their reality through mental processes and arrive at their conclusions through rational thought. From this overly simplistic perspective, it might be argued that infant learning is essentially random and holistic while the adult style tends to be sequential and linear. Yet I believe that a truly holistic model would involve an integration of both learning styles in reconnecting two experiential domains. The difference is that adults have the choice to inhabit either, and it is they who must take the initiative and set the conditions for connection in the 'meeting place.'

As an epilogue to that rejuvenating day with Gail Goldsmith, I remember walking through the main school building after the final shoot of "The Teachable Moment." I was full of enthusiasm and optimism about the message we hoped to deliver. Passing one of the grade one classrooms, I peeked through window in the door and my spirit sank. I saw rows of young children, not much older than our movie stars, sitting stiffly at their desks, eyes forward and pencils in hand while their teacher stood at the front pointing to words on a chart. I walked away with the same feeling I had as a young boy when my Uncle Ralph showed me his collection of butterflies. They were all in a glass case with their delicate wings spread out and pinned to the backboard. I was amazed and horrified. The following day he caught me trying to open up the case with his old penknife. I had no idea that these exquisite creatures were already dead.

CHAPTER FIVE

When Self Meets Other

So far, I have taken an idiosyncratic ramble along the passageways of early childhood, taking many diversions and the occasional 'U-turn' along the way. I realize this might be frustrating for folks who like definitive directions to specified destinations, but I have a different objective in mind. I am more concerned with exploring possibilities than creating yet another theoretical framework, chronological or otherwise, for researchers to investigate and disprove. I fear for our place on this planet and believe our long-term survival now depends upon the realization of our inherent relatedness – to our Selves, each Other and all that surrounds us. This really isn't about saving, or even changing, the world; it's about becoming conscious of our place in the cosmos and aware of our potential to participate in the unfolding of events.

My central hypothesis is that the formula and the resources for change lie within all of us, and our relationships with our children constitute our most effective working laboratory.

In scientific terms my central hypothesis is that the formula and the resources for change lie within all of us, and our relationships with our children constitute our most effective working laboratory. As much as I respect the scientific model, I have neither the time nor the inclination to be bound by the parameters of rigid empirical inquiry. I am unabashedly seeking any evidence I can find to support my stated position while doing whatever I can to set up such laboratories, wherever people are willing and conditions are favorable. I will not be talking about developmental norms, Attention Deficit Disorder and test-tube babies. My concern is with the untapped resources and unrealized potentials that lie at the core of our being and on the periphery of our awareness – our ubiquitous sense of Self. This Self is not the product of psychological development; it is the central motivational and organizational force that can only become known through direct experience. To explicate this further, I will back-track once again and take a closer look at our earliest relational experiences as revealed through the ground-breaking research of Daniel Stern and described in his book, *The Interpersonal World of the Infant,* published in 1985.

A Professor of Psychiatry and Director of the Laboratory of Developmental Processes at Cornell University, Stern developed a set of procedures designed to look beyond conventional theories and assumptions in order to better understand the what infants really experience and feel on the inside. His methods and detailed findings make for fascinating reading but I will take my usual liberties in selectively weaving some of the more general themes and conclusions to support my own perspective.

What I like about Stern's contribution is that his observations lead him to reject the traditional perspective from which human development is seen as a linear trajectory, moving from symbiosis with mother through progressive and discreet stages of separation and individuation. It has been suggested that this model of development was created in the minds of adult males to justify their own relational deficiencies - who am I to argue? Contrary to the party line, Stern's 'observed' infant, almost from birth, possesses a differentiated sense of Self that is seeking both individuation and connection in relationship with the mother. While there is obviously a biological timetable to be respected, the infant's emerging Self is located at the center of the action, organizing internal and external information to explore its own characteristics and potentials through direct involvement with mother. I like this perspective, not only because it fits well with what I've already said, but also because it passes the ultimate test of validity – my own observational and subjective experience. Even at my age, I am still discovering self-limiting aspects within my current relationships that can be traced back to my earliest experiences of being Momma's little boy.

The Infant Self Works from the Inside Out

By the same token, I also appreciate Stern's rejection of traditional 'stage' theory and agree with his assertion that these arbitrary divisions are based more in the mind of the observer than the actual experiences of the infant. From his own observations he concludes that, rather than progressing from one time-limited stage of development to the next, the infant's learning revolves around four distinctive aspects or domains, of the emerging Self. These are …

- The "emergent" Self, refers to the very earliest sense of being, experienced during, or shortly after, birth.

- The "core" Self, relates to the infant's awareness of his or her physical existence and ability to act purposefully – or 'willfully.'

- The "subjective" Self, incorporates a growing awareness of feelings, motives and intentions, giving rise to particular mental states that blend into a cohesive sense of having one's own distinctive inner life.

- The "verbal" Self, enables the infant to make connections between inner states and external circumstances, creating meanings and symbols that can be communicated and shared through the development of language.

Again the thing to keep in mind is that these are not tasks to be completed before the child can move on to the next stage; they are integrated aspects of the Self that continue to create opportunities for awareness and growth throughout the life-span. The implications are that we all have the potential to access our own developmental history and free ourselves from the interruptions and deficits. So far, so good – I can live with all of this.

Every Self needs an Other

But what impresses me most about Stern's work is its relational focus. Throughout his investigation, he pays particular attention to how each aspect of the developing Self is reflected and expressed through the infant's on going relationship with the mother. In this sense the categories of 'emergence,' 'core,' 'subjective,' and 'verbal,' apply to the developing relationship as much as they apply to the emergence of the Self. This serves to underscore my fundamental position that, from our earliest awareness of our existence on this planet, the inseparable duality of Self and Other is the essential dynamic that makes us human. In this sense we are our relationships,

From our earliest awareness of our existence on this planet, the inseparable duality of Self and Other is the essential dynamic that makes us human.

and whatever we do in our minds to detach one from the other can only serve to arrest our individual and collective development. In my view, we can no longer afford to consider this as just another intellectual proposition. This is a notion that can only be fully grasped experientially and that means incorporating it into the way we conduct our lives and, in particular, the way we relate to our children. As always, this is a choice we can only make for our Selves.

Obviously there is a sequential aspect to Stern's perspective – that's what the term 'development' means – but it's not the same time-ordered progression advocated by the traditional stage theorists. In effect Stern's research affirms what many parents already know – that an infant's emerging sense of Self is expressed through unpredictable leaps and bounds. Parents frequently report that, following each of these surges, they suddenly find themselves dealing with a different person, and in a way they are. According to Stern, these shifts are most likely to occur between 0-2 months, 2-7 months, 9-15 months and 18-30 months but there are no guarantees. The developmental process involves all four domains interacting with the external world and infants will integrate this experience in their own time and their own way. If pressed to respond according to

Adults who possess a secure sense of Self will intuitively support this natural process and delight in each new expression of the young Self as it sets out to establish its unique presence in the world.

specific criteria and a fixed time schedule, the natural development of the Self will become stifled. The infant Self learns 'holistically,' employing all of the senses to take in and integrate new information from many sources – inside and outside. Adults who possess a secure sense of Self will intuitively support this natural process and delight in each new expression of the young Self as it sets out to establish its unique presence in the world. This is a Self with the potential to carve out its own pathway, through childhood and beyond.

On the other side of the coin, the idea that past experiences continue to interact with the present also implies that early injuries may continue to impact the emergence of the whole. After many years of working with adult couples I don't need to be convinced that recurring relationship difficulties can often be traced back to what happened, or didn't happen, in the earliest formative years. When these interruptions are 'triggered,' they are played out as real-life experiences and usually attributed to circumstances within current relationships. Unless the original injury is identified and addressed, it will continue to find a way through regardless of the circumstances. The good news particularly for therapists, is that such interruptions can usually be accessed later in life and resolved in the present through the intrinsic resources of the Self.

No Child Should be Expected to be 'Normal'

Thankfully one of the casualties of Stern's model is the revered concept of the developmental 'norm'. Since we can never be sure what a particular child is, or should be, learning at any point in time, the imposition of performance goals and achievement markers makes absolutely no sense. In fact, such expectations can be injurious to the developing Self, particularly when communicated through the minds, morals and motives of proud and pushy parents. In my

Few factors have wrought more damage on a fledgling Self than the pressures applied by concerned parents who want their kids to be ahead of the game from the get-go.

professional experience, few factors have wrought more damage on a fledgling Self than the pressures applied by concerned parents who want their kids to be ahead of the game from the get-go. In such cases the inherent value and integrity of the Self is sacrificed to the gods of a competitive, achievement-oriented society – a world of winners and losers. "I want the best for him," they say, or "We need to get her into a 'Head-Start' program." The tragedy is that such parents are delighted when the educational system takes over where they left off, and even national programs purporting to be in the 'best interests' of all children operate under such banners as "no child left behind". If we cannot produce a generation of children capable of competing with the Chinese for the new international markets, we are surely doomed. Forgive them, Lord, for they know not what they do.

Parenting is Not a Separate Task

Actually, there's not that much for parents to do. I realize this line will not go down well with folks who find themselves struggling to fit childcare into an already complex and demanding schedule. For what it's worth, over the years I've faced countless confrontations with irate parents on this issue. As much as I can empathize with their plight, I still maintain that most of the pressure stems from a cultural attitude that considers parenting to be a separate responsibility, a task unto itself. Of course it's easy for me to babble on about how remote tribes manage to incorporate the responsibilities of parenting into their everyday lives and offer their children opportunities to participate. I do understand that life in the jungle of Montreal is very different from life in the Amazon Basin, but we always have the option to modify our attitudes and behaviors. Having chosen to abandon the old model of the nuclear family, the onus is now upon us to find other ways to include our kids in our alternative lifestyles. If we don't want them, we can simply choose not to have them.

When we make a conscious choice to become parents, our central responsibility is to understand our reasons along with the far-reaching implications of our decision. In this case, the chances are we will be able to offer unconditional caring, empathy and love, and the Self we have taken under our wings will have all it requires to set out on its own voyage of discovery. If we are able to suspend our own agendas, we can begin to understand that, at the core, children already know what we know and seek only to create their own place in the world through our support and guidance. Children need to be known as much as they want to know, and our curiosity about them is as important as our willingness to hold them in our arms, change their diapers and show them how to tie their shoe laces.

The Infant Self is an Opportunist

Stern's work offers impressive evidence to show how, given the security of effective caring and unconditional love, babies know exactly what they want and are quite capable of communicating their needs and preferences. As inherently social beings, their natural desire is to learn how to be with other social beings, and by nature's design, the tuned-in parent doesn't require a prescription and a logbook to decide what to do next. Infants live in the 'eternal moment'; they don't reflect upon the past and anticipate the future like adults. The key to effective parenting is more about the ability to respond to the child in

Children need to be known as much as they want to know, and our curiosity about them is as important as our willingness to hold them in our arms, change their diapers and show them how to tie their shoe laces.

the moment than in taking responsibility for what the future may have in store. From the 'gaze' onwards, infants seek to establish their own self-regulation, not by responding to mother giving up control, but by actively taking control on their own behalf. On the other side, mother serves as a 'self-regulating other', constantly adjusting her responses to maintain levels of external stimulation the infant can tolerate. In this delicate relational equation, mother brings her intuition, wisdom and history while the infant

The key to effective parenting is more about the ability to respond to the child in the moment than in taking respon-sibility for what the future may have in store.

brings the gifts of immediacy and spontaneity. Described analytically, this may appear as a subtle and complex process – and it is. In the experience of mother and child, and seen through the eyes of an intuitive observer, it is readily accepted as a perfectly natural and taken-for-granted way of being.

Becoming Me, Without Losing You

What clearly distinguishes Stern's analysis from that of previous investigators is his picture of early development as a constant vacillation between separation and connection. In this he rejects the 'object relations' view that the infant begins the developmental journey in an undifferentiated, or symbiotic, merger with mother. While he does not say that separation and attachment difficulties may relate more to the unmet needs of the mother than the current needs of child, the inference is there for the taking. For me, this reflects a major deficit in Stern's overall perspective. For his stance to be truly 'relational,' he would be compelled to give equal attention to the subjective experiences of both mother and infant in exploring

*Separation and attach-
ment difficulties may
relate more to the
unmet needs of the
mother than the
current needs of child.*

whatever is happening between them. Nevertheless, his basic propositions not only reformulate the entire nature and spectrum of the developmental process but also, to my mind at least, provide a sound empirical foundation for exploring the arena we refer to as 'transitional space.' I could easily spend the remainder of this chapter speculating about the implications, but will limit myself to the proposition that, what the infant actually experiences is not a passive world of disconnected and impersonal objects but an arena constantly stirred by internal and external personal activity and interpersonal encounters. In other words the 'meeting place' is open for business from the moment mother and child make their first eye-to-eye connection.

At this point according to Stern, the emerging Self of the infant is already actively receiving and organizing information that initiates and elaborates the sensual domain of the core self. This activity subsequently opens up the social realm of the subjective self and so on. As each domain is activated and elaborated, it becomes integrated into an expanding whole, and the infant responds with increasing coherence and purpose. Throughout this process the necessary pre-condition is the infant's sense of security, derived from being cared for by a consistent and loving presence. If mother is not physically and energetically available or, her own needs dominate those of her child, the delicate balance of their relationship is disrupted

*If mother is not
physically and energy-
etically available or, her
own needs dominate
those of her child, the
delicate balance of their
relationship is dis-
rupted and the devel-
opmental pathway is
effectively blocked.*

and the developmental pathway is effectively blocked. Since all domains are open and active it is impossible to know from the outside which particular aspect of the infant Self actually experiences the interruption.

We are talking about the early development of an integrated and complex experiential system, and if the problem persists it is likely to have a significant impact on the system as a whole. Deprived of the essential life-affirming bond, the infant has nowhere to go and faced with the terrifying prospect of abandonment, regresses to the most primal need on the developmental continuum – physical survival. In this cause he or she will readily sacrifice all other needs to ensure that the external life support system is in place and working effectively. In this critical reversal of the natural sequence, the roles of mother and child may undergo an inversion through which the child is coerced into becoming the consistent, caring and loving regulatory presence, attending to the needs of the mother. In this way the fledgling Self is stripped of its own volition and drawn into the service of the caring other – the state Jack Rosenberg refers to as "agency." Taken to the extreme, this might seem like a far-fetched and remote possibility, but I would go so far as to suggest that, to some extent, this dynamic can be found in most mother-child relationships. Within my own life I am constantly reminded of how my early failures to make 'Mommy' happy continue to influence my relationships with others.

You won't find this discussion and conclusion in Stern's book, but as I warned you earlier, I have no scruples about selectively blending what others have said into my own theories. This does not however, include distorting or deliberately manipulating the evidence, and I make every effort to ensure that the essence of borrowed content remains acknowledged, explicit and uncompromised. In this instance my purpose is to identify interruptions to the emerging Self that might inhibit its overall development and volition.

The Three Basic Developmental Needs

As it stands, Stern's work offers solid support for my assertion that babies are social beings seeking to take charge of their lives in their connection with others. His 'connection-separation' model also endorses my belief that healthy development is brought about through an intricate interaction among three fundamental variables. The first is the consistent presence of a primary bond in which the infant feels secure, loved and cared for within one special relationship. On the other side is the degree of freedom, or breathing room, that allows the child to make self-directed choices with support and encouragement. The delicate balance between connection and separation is established by the quality of empathic attunement within the mother-child relationship. Specifically this refers to the ability of the primary caretaker to accurately sense and respond to, the subjective experiences of the child. While I appreciate much of what Stern has to say about these three relational arenas, his predominantly psychoanalytic view leaves his 'observed infant' significantly less unique and self-directed than my own thesis would suggest. With this in mind I would like to review these three arenas in more detail.

1. Bonding

From the evidence presented, it seems clear that our earliest relationship with mother establishes the foundation for our emerging sense of Self and becomes the blueprint for future relationships. Children nurtured in a caring and loving way are assured of their inherent 'rightness,' and set out on the human trail with confidence. Early developmental interruptions occur when, for whatever reason, mother is unable to provide this consistent, loving presence. Occasional lapses in connection are easily accommodated by the infant and may actually serve to enhance the individuation process. In circumstances where the security of the bond is made conditional upon the infant's behavior, the functional and expressive needs of the developing Self are sacrificed in the service of survival. Severe developmental injuries occur when mother is physically or emotionally absent for extended periods of time, leaving the child to face the terrifying prospects of abandonment and annihilation. Such injuries are exacerbated when neglect is combined with physical or emotional abuse, and children who begin life in this way are likely to end up in one kind of institution or another. While working in residential treatment settings, I came to recognize severe early bonding injuries through one pervasive and enduring characteristic – the absence of empathy, conscience and guilt. In accordance with Stern's view that all stages of development remain accessible throughout the life span, I became convinced that the only effective 'treatment' is to recreate the conditions of the primary bond, using a childcare specialist as a surrogate parent. As you might imagine, this is a very demanding and time consuming task, but I was fortunate to be working with skilled and dedicated child and youth care workers who were willing to push themselves beyond the comfortable parameters of their professional skills and personal resources. Thanks to them,

> *Severe developmental injuries occur when mother is physically or emotionally absent for extended periods of time, leaving the child to face the terrifying prospects of abandonment and annihilation ... children who begin life in this way are likely to end up in one kind of institution or another.*

a small group of children rediscovered their connection with themselves and others and are now leading self-responsible relational lives. I don't need follow-up data to inform me that, in some cases, our efforts did not appear successful but that's par for the course. On the other hand, the workers relished the opportunity to explore new territory and expressed no regrets about having tried. For my own part, my role as program director made it possible for me to protect them from a system that demands simplistic prescriptions for cost effective outcomes.

Sadly, to the best of my knowledge, there are no documented examples of this approach being used elsewhere. For the most part, early bonding injuries are not recognized and children who carry this deficit are subjected to the usual range of psychological and pharmacological interventions. In many cases, traditional cognitive and behavioral methods appear to be effective on the surface but such outcomes are simply reflections of a disconnected Self that is struggling to survive in a cold and impersonal world. These youngsters regard others as objects to be manipulated and deceived in a cold-blooded game of power and control. Their superficial compliance and contrived authenticity are learned behaviors designed to keep the world distant and submissive. Sooner or later however, the early injury will manifest through the façade in the form of callous actions carried out with no compunction or subsequent remorse. The consequences for such actions whether lenient or punishing, have little impact other than to provide more information in the quest for future gratification. In treatment settings, such youngsters are usually tagged with the 'psychopathic

Unless the bonding injury is successfully addressed, these imprisoned souls remain as a danger to themselves and more particularly, to others.

personality' label and eventually pronounced 'untreatable.' Much as I have always resisted the classifications of psychopathology, I have to acknowledge that unless the bonding injury is successfully addressed, these imprisoned souls remain as a danger to themselves and more particularly, to others.

THE MYSTERY OF THE MISSING NINE MONTHS

While most developmental theorists make the assumption that bonding begins at birth, the evidence now clearly suggests that the process begins much earlier – from the point of conception. This would explain Stern's observation that newborns appear to possess an innate ability to act on their own behalf (self-agency), a sense of their own continuity (self-history), and experience a broad range of feeling and emotional states (self-affectivity). These are the essential indications of a separate and purposeful Self. This is not the cognitively constructed Self that comes from systematic learning but an undeniable sense of being, drawn from internal bio-energetic experiences and external conditions. This then becomes the foundation, the essence from which the newborn will begin to create his or her defined place in the world. If this is the case, we are obliged to recognize that the bond is created in the period between conception and birth and understand why the physical separation of mother is such a momentous event.

THE CHILD AS SPIRIT

Whatever takes place between a mother and her unborn child, there is one fundamental question that virtually all theorists, including Stern, have chosen to ignore. What is the essential nature of the 'organism' that begins with the merger of ovum and sperm and (hopefully) ends up in mother's arms? Are we talking about a spiritual entity assuming a human form, or a biological creature

Are we talking about a spiritual entity assuming a human form, or a biological creature conforming to its genetic heritage and imperatives?

conforming to its genetic heritage and imperatives? In that first moment of contact do mother and child meet 'I' to 'I' or simply 'eye' to 'eye'? Our answer to this question makes a huge difference to the way we regard children, and the way we see ourselves. If you were to conduct a survey, I'm convinced the vast majority of respondents would opt for the former yet our rational cognitive minds are much more at ease with the latter.

If we choose to remove the spiritual being from the human being, we are left to define ourselves accordingly. Within the scientific paradigm our biological developmental can be accounted for through Darwinian Evolutionism. In this framework the emergence of human consciousness is seen to be the product of biologically programmed neo-cortical development with no place for the creativity, unpredictability and power of the human will. This 'soul-less' stance implies that the infant's contribution to the bonding process is no more than a response to some unknown biological program with the emerging Self as a cognitive overlay constructed from the cues presented by others, particularly the mother. However you wish to look at it, the bio-cognitive model presents a fundamentally deterministic stance. This I have chosen to reject.

Within the 'scientific' traditions of developmental psychology, Stern probably goes further than anybody in entertaining the possibility that we are the co-creators of our first relationship, but for my money his 'observed infant' remains bound and gagged in a biological, cognitive and psychoanalytic straightjacket. So when we talk about newborns as active participants in the bonding process, we can only conclude that they are seeking to satisfy their basic physiological needs and that the only purpose of the infant self is to organize and integrate internal and external experience to that end. Since the self of the mother operates in the same way, their relationship can be conceptualized as a complex system of mutual information processing. Even the Star Wars robots C3PO and R2D2 had more going for them than this.

I have already articulated my belief that the authentic Self is a deeply rooted feeling state that reflects our unique essence, so I will try not to belabor the point. But just to remind you, this felt sense is neither biological nor cognitive at the core, although these systems are certainly involved in its expression and elaboration. Its essence is spiritual, its substance is energetic, and its central location is in the body. It is not a creation of the mind but the kernel from which our consciousness continually expands. If this still seems irrational or unscientific, I would repeat my earlier suggestion that you take a look at Danah Zoher's book *The Quantum Self*. If you choose to reject the whole idea I would urge you to delve into the wisdom of your subjectivity and create your own alternative. The only other course is to accept that you are, and always will be, the product of forces beyond your understanding and control.

> The authentic Self is a deeply rooted feeling state … Its essence is spiritual, its substance is energetic, and its central location is in the body.

Returning to the matter of primary bonding, I want to consider the implications of insinuating an essence of Self that is spiritual in nature, energetic in substance and purposeful in design. Call me a romantic but I find it hard to believe that anyone who has witnessed an infant 'gazing' into the eyes of a devoted mother would be left

At the heart of the matter, the Self, the real Self, is pursuing its most enduring objective – to see and be seen, by an Other.

unmoved at the deepest level. This is not a prelude to action; it is an event complete unto itself. Look into the eyes of the infant. Is this the expression of a child desperately seeking some form of service? Look into the eyes of the mother. Is this a woman preparing to offer such a service? Some romantics see a couple 'in love,' but what I sense is a re-connection of two Selves that have traveled together along the most arduous leg of the human adventure and now rest in each other's eyes. When people attempt to describe this moment, using terms like 'sensory discrimination' and 'proprioceptive feedback,' I recoil in horror. It may well be that the infant brain is rehearsing its role by learning how to classify facial features and respond to sensory cues, but this is secondary information. At the heart of the matter, the Self, the *real* Self, is pursuing its most enduring objective – to see and be seen, by an Other. If I were to insert my own dialogue into the scenario, it would be something like "So, here I am and there you are."

BONDING IS AN ENERGETIC AFFAIR

Despite its centrality to the pure science of physics, western psychology and medicine have generally resisted incorporating energy into their working models of human life. Perhaps this has something to do with its ubiquitous and unobservable nature but there can be no denying that we are all energetic beings living in an energetically charged universe. Until recently, science relied upon the optical microscope to examine the structure of matter and expose the incredibly complex workings of biological organisms. However, if you were to take a look at your body using an electron microscope, you would see constantly shifting patterns of particles and waves randomly transforming from one to the other - the energetic improvisations of your life. While the shifts may appear chaotic and unpredictable, closer study will reveal repetitive configurations or themes – melodies embedded in countless octaves within the cosmic symphony. Some of these melodies may reflect enduring genetic and situational variations, but if cell biologist Bruce Lipton is correct, there is one central voice – a conductor if you like – that interprets, co-ordinates and shapes the whole. Here in this unexplored and unpredictable quantum world, we find the human Self in its most essential energetic form, as a unique configuration of particles and waves drawing together an individual human life, from the unfolding of consciousness to the pain in the big toe on the left foot.

Just as the core Self creates its own distinctive energetic spectrum, so the individual exists within an energetic field.

Just as the core Self creates its own distinctive energetic spectrum, so the individual exists within an energetic field shared by other energetic beings. When a mother holds her baby against her heart, the infant's heart responds – communion and harmony that forms the energetic nucleus of all bonded relationships. When this occurs, both Selves are changed in some way and the story of their encounter becomes written into the universal energetic script. In the Quantum world this same phenomenon has been observed in the pairing of photons – the most elementary sub-atomic particles. Once the pairing is established, each photon remains 'in touch' with the other even when separated by vast distances across time and space. Without giving any thought to the complexities of quantum mechanics, my partner Judith drew upon her intuition to write in her journal:

Somewhere between desire and death
Two lost souls met
And found themselves in one another
Never to be the same again

If such connections can occur between one human being and another, where else are they more likely to take place than in the exquisite wordless encounters between a mother and her newborn child?

I realize that, for many traditionalists, this is too much to take, but I suspect their major discomfort arises more from the methodological implications than any challenge to their personal world-views. From the ingenuity of the most elementary machines to the sophisticated technology of space flight, scientists have been harnessing, generating and measuring the raw energy of the universe for centuries. The transformed energy of life, with all its subtleties and variations is a very different matter. In this regard the family dog is much better equipped to sense the energy of human emotions and intentions than even the most sophisticated mechanical sensors. When it comes to resonating with the complex energetic spectrum of a human being, there is only one instrument capable of the task – the full energetic sensorium of another human being. Unfortunately we have pronounced this instrument to be irrational, untrustworthy, and distinctly unscientific. Hardly a day went by in graduate school when I wasn't reminded of this dictum. Information gleaned through the senses was sometimes permitted in terms of visual, auditory and olfactory cues but any suggestion of intuitive or energetic sensing among human beings was to be scoffed at.

BONDING VERSUS 'ATTACHMENT'

Before moving on I want to make a clear distinction between my version of bonding and what has become known as Attachment Theory; a perspective that has dominated developmental theories and psychological practices over the past decade or so. On the surface it might appear that its basis premises are similar to my own – particularly its central assumption that our adult styles of relating are shaped by our earliest relational experiences. My decision to detach myself from attachment theory is not an attempt to make me right and others wrong; it's only a way to clarify my own position. Allow me to explain.

Attachment Theory was originated by the British psychiatrist John Bowlby in the early 1990's and arose from his curiosity about the distress exhibited by infants who had been separated from their primary caretaker. As a psychoanalyst influenced by Darwin's theories of evolution, he concluded that attachment-seeking behaviors such as crying, clinging and searching are adaptive responses common to all mammalian offspring in the quest for survival. Zoologist Conrad Lorenze supported this view and noted how human infant social behavior seemed to resemble that displayed by our primate cousins, including emotional expressions and attachment seeking. In the 1950's animal researchers Harlow and Zimmerman demonstrated how Rhesus Monkeys displayed a distinct preference for a terry-cloth surrogate 'mother' over a wire mesh version, even when only the latter provided food. At the most basic level animal researchers observed how fledgling birds instinctively follow their keepers around the farmyard – a behavioral response known as 'imprinting.' The common consensus was that we are all locked into a biological program designed to ensure our physical survival.

Working from the assumption that human attachment behaviors reflect a complex form of imprinting, Mary Ainsworth, a colleague of John Bowlby, developed a laboratory method for studying infant responses to being separated from the mother. These responses were grouped into three general categories – 'Secure'; 'Anxious Resistant'; and 'Avoidant.' Mary Ainsworth had finally given researchers something to observe and measure in an arena that had hitherto remained obscure and almost untouchable – the relational dynamics of early childhood. Now it was possible for researchers to demonstrate how an infant's responses to separation anxiety evolve into particular patterns or styles that subsequently play themselves out in their adult lives.

There were brand new 'disorders' to work with and an enthusiastic group of early childhood specialists, notably Robert Zaslow in California and Foster Cline at the Attachment Center in Evergreen, Colorado. Their underlying assumption was that the child was consumed with suppressed rage, which needed to be released by the caretaker or surrogate. Their methods were designed to induce this bottled up anger through direct confrontation and physical restraint. During the catharsis the child would be held firmly, even lain upon until he or she 'capitulated,' often breaking down into sobs. Having gained control the therapist would respond warmly to the child, thereby creating a new level of trust that could be transferred into the relationship with parent or primary caretaker. In the follow up programs, caretakers were taught a variety of obedience training techniques designed to punish willful non-compliance and reinforce the desired attachment behaviors.

It doesn't take much insight to appreciate the damage such coercive methods might inflict upon a fragile and fearful Self seeking to find its place in the world, or how submission to external authority would effectively quash any sense of personal autonomy. Obviously these were not considered to be matters of concern by therapists seeking appropriate attachment behaviors, or the caretakers who wanted to be loved and obeyed without having to acknowledge their part in the relational breakdown. Yet, for whatever reason, such methods continued to flourish. As Foster Cline pointed out in his 1992 publication *Hope for*

High Risk and Rage Filled Children, even the renowned
'humanistic' psychiatrist Milton Erickson was known to
have advised a mother to sit on her non compliant son for
hours at a time. In addition he suggested she feed him
with cold oatmeal while she and her daughter enjoyed
appetizing food. According to Erickson's own reports, the
child did indeed become more compliant and even
trembled when his mother looked at him. Case closed.

In 1972 Robert Zaslow was brought before the
Psychological Examining Committee of the Board of
Medical Examiners in California and condemned for his
inhuman practices. In a 2006 report commissioned by the
American Professional Society on the Abuse of Children,
Attachment Therapy was severely criticized for its theory,
methodology and research claims. In the face of such
concerns the overall theory was refined to emphasize
attachment as a two-way relational issue, and rather than
attempting to force children into loving their parents,
practitioners began to stress caretaker sensitivity and
'positive regard.' For this we – and many isolated children
- should be eternally grateful.

I recognize that many practitioners who continue to
practice under the banner of 'attachment-based' therapy,
now talk about our ability to change our relational patterns
through self-awareness and it may well be that some are
no longer tied to the biological roots of their tradition - at
least not consciously. Yet I continue to question the
underlying assumptions of the new 'attachment-based'
therapies, along with their diagnostic models and
treatment practices. I still shudder whenever references are
made to "Attachment Disorders" and "Reactive
Attachment Disorders" as listed in the Diagnostic and
Statistical Manual of Mental Disorders" (DSM 1V).

2. Breathing Room

The quality of the bond with mother determines the degree to which the infant feels connected, safe and cared for. Interruptions in the bonding process are transitory confrontations with the Nemo that may threaten the child's sense of security and evoke the universal fear of abandonment. On the other hand, brief interruptions are not only inevitable, but also necessary for the fledgling Self to begin the work of carving out its own unique place in the world. In other words the infant needs both bonding and breathing room.

The relationship between these two subjective experiences is a delicate balance that cannot be established through some *a priori* parenting prescription. It is an arrangement that must be sensed energetically and negotiated intuitively between the parties involved. If bonding interruptions are extreme, the fearful infant will clamor for contact with mother in the interests of survival. Conversely, if mother is overly possessive or protective, the infant has no place to go and the Self becomes stifled. All babies will experience both these conditions to some degree but given the opportunity, they will gradually take charge of the process by moving closer when they need connection and further away when they need personal space. In my experience, there's nothing more delightful than watching a contented, Self-directed baby exploring the physical world while mother smiles and waits patiently for the homecoming. As the Self becomes more defined and central in the developmental progression, it becomes

There is nothing more delightful than watching a contented, Self-directed baby exploring the physical world while mother smiles and waits patiently for the homecoming.

increasingly capable of replacing mother as the place of safety and well being. To use a crude sporting analogy, the Self gradually becomes the home base in the relational ball game. In adulthood a person who is able to move freely between Self and Other with confidence and integrity, operates within the highest level of the developmental continuum – relational autonomy.

NOT TOO CLOSE AND NOT TOO FAR

However successful we become in managing our relational affairs, our earliest fears of abandonment and inundation continue to find their way into our dealings with the world. In his books *Body, Self & Soul, and The Intimate Couple*, Jack Rosenberg and his colleagues clearly outline how our individual defensive patterns, and much of what we call 'personality,' are actually repetitive manifestations of our earliest attempts to deal with these sources of anxiety. Because this learning takes place prior to the development of our cognitive faculties, its location is cellular rather than cerebral. For this reason, it cannot be conveniently modified or eradicated psychologically through insight followed by cognitive and behavioral adjustments. The best we can do is to recognize the source and the nature of our anxiety and return to the business of our lives as quickly and effectively as possible. I will discuss the implications of this in more detail later.

Given a secure bond with mother, breathing room enables the infant Self to explore its own volition in its own time and in its own way. Such infants are granted permission to have their own thoughts and feelings while making their own choices and mistakes. What they require more than anything is a mirror – an opportunity to be recognized as a separate entity in the world with its own purposes and internal experiences. The ability to offer a mirror that accurately matches a child's inside experience is an indispensable parenting skill that will be discussed at

*Children who are
fortunate enough
to have a secure
connection with others,
the freedom to act on
their own behalf and
an accurate mirror to
reflect the substance of
their experience, walk
firmly on the pathway
toward self-fulfillment
and self-responsibility.*

length later in this chapter. Meanwhile, I want to underscore the assertion that children who are fortunate enough to have a secure connection with others, the freedom to act on their own behalf and an accurate mirror to reflect the substance of their experience, walk firmly on the pathway toward self-fulfillment and self-responsibility. With continued support along the way, it's highly unlikely they will ever fall into the traps of helplessness and victim-hood, holding others responsible for their happiness and personal choices. In contrast, the child with inundating parents will have difficulty establishing a separate sense of Self and will generally avoid intimacy in future relationships for fear of being controlled and overwhelmed. Here again we are talking about the art of 'good enough' parenting.

The inability or unwillingness to provide sufficient breathing room is often considered to be the pitfall of the over protective and devoted parent. In the western world, this stems from a cultural prescription that 'good parents' should care for their children by attending to their every need. As I have said many times, and in many different ways, most of the difficulties arise unwittingly from the interruptions to the parent's own developmental history. If mother's early bonding brought fears of abandonment, the chances are she will hang onto her child as a replacement love-object. Alternatively, a mother who experienced significant early inundation may come to resent the demands of the infant and distance herself more than the infant is able to tolerate. This creates the potential for two equally disturbing outcomes. The most obvious is that the child will become increasingly demanding and the mother's resentment will turn into anger and possible neglect or abuse. The other is that the infant will simply give up and manifest a condition known as 'failure to thrive'.

I mention these themes only as possibilities of which there are many subtle variations. An inundated mother for example, may also inundate rather than abandon the infant in an attempt to replace those parts of the Self that were taken away. Similarly a mother who experienced early abandonment may remain distant, rather than face the prospect of being abandoned in yet another primary relationship. Either way the probability is strengthened by our natural tendency to parent as we ourselves were parented. While there is no doubt that unresolved early developmental injuries are passed down from one generation to the next, it is impossible to predict how they will manifest themselves in any particular mother-child relationship. For this, the information we need can only be derived from one source – the subjective experience of both parties.

In the most general sense, bonding and breathing room are components within a single equation in which the quality of the bond is always the central variable. It isn't a question of one or the other, but the balance between the two. In the rare and extreme case, a mother who has never had the benefit of an effective primary bond, has no way of relating to her child as a connected, yet separate human being and the issue of breathing room is never brought into the equation. These are the tragic circumstances resulting in the severe developmental injuries that eventually manifest themselves in the child as the condition I referred to earlier as the 'psychopathic personality.' There is only one resolution to this calamity; somehow mother must find a way to repair her own bonding injury. Even if this were possible, however, the chances are it would be too late to re-direct the developmental career of the deprived infant. Much as I believe in the cause of preserving the sacred relationship between a mother and her child, I have no hesitation in declaring that, in such circumstances, the baby should be removed and placed with surrogate parents with the least possible distress to both parties.

3. Energetic Attunement

In the present context, 'energetic attunement' refers to a mother's ability to find that delicate balance between bonding and breathing room by sensing and responding to her infant's internal feelings and desires. At the most basic level, she understands when her child is feeling contented, distressed, inundated or abandoned. Since bonding is very much a two-way arrangement, this implies that the infant is also able to sense and respond to changes in mother's internal states. When both are happy, this may appear as a playful mime with each performer imitating the other and finding pleasure in their synchronicity. However, if you look deeper, you will see their exchanges as a delicate dance in which each partner responds to the steps of the other, each contributing subtle variations to the tempo and intensity of the encounter. If you really want to understand what's going on, you must take a deep breath and tune into the energy channel. Then what you see through your eyes and hear through your ears will be distilled through your senses and you will find yourself moving to the same rhythm as the dancers. You will become a participant-observer, albeit from a respectful and non-intrusive distance, engaged in a lived-in experience. In short you will have invoked the most sensitive and powerful observation instrument of all – your core energetic Self.

It's important to understand that these energetic encounters between a mother and her baby are not the means to some pre-determined developmental end – they are complete experiential events that celebrate the simple communion of being together, whether in joy or in sadness. In their sharing each becomes a mirror for the other in the most open and authentic way. Of course there will be times when mother's internal state does not match that of her young partner. This is not necessarily a breakdown in attunement. As long they remain energetically available to one another this offers the child an opportunity to experience himself or herself as a separate being. Such discrepancies can also be re-assuring – "Everything is okay my little one. There's nothing to be afraid of, mother is here."

As the child's cognitive abilities come more into play and mother steps back to see her child as a separate thinking, feeling and acting being, this spontaneous mutuality begins to diminish. The focus of their relationship shifts from unmediated intuition to inferences drawn from external cues and 'knowing' becomes an understanding based upon past experience. This does not mean that the 'intuitive' aspects of the relationship are lost forever, only that they are contained while other developmental imperatives take up the space. Unfortunately, our involvement in a highly cognitive and competitive world of ambition and achievement can suppress this profound level of 'knowing,' but it remains available whenever the channel is opened. How many stories have you heard about a mother who is suddenly overcome with an overwhelming sense that her adult son or daughter is in trouble in some distant place? To the rational mind, such accounts seem unbelievable, yet we all know they are undeniably true.

> *Unfortunately, our involvement in a highly cognitive and competitive world of ambition and achievement can suppress this profound level of 'knowing'.*

SELF-BOUNDARIES AND ATTUNEMENT

As the child's Self becomes more differentiated and cognitively understood, it's energetic emanations become increasingly varied and complex. This energy moves out beyond the skin to create its own unique vibrations in the world. The energy of the integrated Self does not simply dissipate into the ether, it remains contained within its own parameters, defining the Self as a distinct entity. This makes it possible for the emerging Self to make contact with Others without losing its own internal integrity. These parameters are not fixed or rigid, they are in constant motion responding the individual's internal states and external conditions. They operate much like a jellyfish sensing its way through the ocean. For two integrated Selves to make full energetic contact their individual parameters or boundaries, they must be recognized and above all, respected.

While the infant Self has always possessed its own energetic boundaries, attunement now requires a full appreciation of the individual as an individuating human being. This is a shift that the attuned mother will naturally accommodate, but whenever two adult strangers come together to create a close or intimate relationship they face a formidable challenge. The energy of the energetic Self is now surrounded by a complex array of psychological and behavioral 'stuff' that serves to express or protect its core essence. This is why enduring intimate relationships between adults are so difficult to create and sustain. It might even be argued that this is the greatest challenge that life puts before us. The only real assurance we have is that, at the deepest level, the energetic connection between mother and child is present in all human relationships. All we really have to do is to hang out at the contact boundary and rediscover what makes us all human and connected. If all this seems a little mystical or abstract don't be too concerned. I will ground these images in observable reality as the story unfolds.

As adults, our relationships are profoundly influence by our earliest experiences of attunement with our primary caretaker. This lays the foundation for our ability to remain open to ourselves and empathic toward others – critical ingredients of any close and meaningful relationship. However, nobody can claim to move into adulthood as a fully open and empathic human being. We all have our deceptions, deflections and defenses and these must be acknowledged and addressed before we can move on. The primary vehicle for change can be as simple as taking a breath, recognizing the sensations in the body and letting go of the stifled energy. This can also be a shared experience of attunement. The next time you make love without engaging your mind, notice how in those ecstatic moments of mutuality, your energy and breath are synchronized with those of your partner. If this is not the case – better luck next time.

> *This lays the foundation for our ability to remain open to ourselves and empathic toward others – critical ingredients of any close and meaningful relationship.*

GLOBAL ATTUNEMENT

At the broadest level, I do not believe we will survive as a species unless we become energetically attuned to each other and ourselves, no matter how much thought we give to our plight. If we refuse to acknowledge our energetic nature or fail to understand its centrality in our relatedness, even between a mother and her baby, then our alienation will surely lead us into extinction. The most we can hope for is some form of planetary crisis that will literally shake us into our senses before all is lost. If this is inevitable, I would echo the exhortation of George W. Bush

– "Bring it on!" If not then perhaps we can try to clean up our own lives and our relationships, particularly with our children, and with at least the same dedication we might give to recycling our Pepsi-Cola bottles.

THE SELF IN THE MIRROR

The ability to accurately mirror the experience of another is the product of energetic and empathetic attunement. Since most developmental theorists regard the Self as a mental construct, the need to be mirrored is generally considered to arise after the first year of life. If you choose to believe babies come into this world with a sense of Self, the immediate availability of a mirror becomes central to the process of individuation and separation. Fortunately babies are considerably smarter than the experts and do their best to draw us into providing the mirror they need. I have already discussed how adults seem to know intuitively how to respond with appropriate gestures and expressions, but the key to understanding mirroring with pre-verbal infants is to recognize that the process is fundamentally energetic. The baby is not responding to words or gestures but to the energetic feeling tone received from the other. Such a mirror provides the infant Self with two essential validating ingredients. In the first place it confirms his or her existence in the world as a separate and unique human being. Secondly it offers a gentle assurance that internal experiences are real and significant. Without this foundation the cognitive overlays of the Self will always be plagued by uncertainty, hanging on to fragile self-images and seeking external assurances.

The key to understanding mirroring with pre-verbal infants is to recognize that the process is fundamentally energetic.

Whether we are aware of it or not, infants will seek their own reflection through their primary relationships. I have used the term 'accurate mirroring' to describe circumstances in which the significant adults are able to sense and reflect the child's internal experiences. Again this is not about establishing a perfect match and reasonable degrees of slippage give permission for the infant to be different from the presented image. If the mirror is persistently inaccurate, vague or otherwise distorted, however, the child's sense of Self is similarly compromised. This is what Otto Rank referred to "faulty mirroring." During infancy this applies particularly to inaccurate or inadequate reflections of the child's emotional world of hurts, frustrations, joys and excitement. In the energetic realm these can only be effectively mirrored through corresponding authentic responses experienced and expressed by the Other. In a sense the child is saying: "I will know my feelings are real and valid when I know you are feeling the same way. If you don't recognize my feelings, they cannot be important. If your feelings are always different from mine, I will give up mine and adopt yours."

Whatever the experts have to say, I believe most mirroring injuries occur during the first three months following birth, and for this reason they are generally difficult to identify and remediate later. Left as they are, they continue to compromise the integrity of the Self and eventually become incorporated into the legacies handed down from one generation to the next. Although such mirroring deficiencies may take on a variety of idiosyncratic forms, it might be useful to exemplify them by using some broad and general categories. Please don't let frivolous quotations distract you from the serious nature of these mis-attunements.

The term 'over-mirroring' is used to describe an adult's attempts to influence a child's experience by inflating or amplifying the reflections. With verbal children this often takes the form of exaggerated responses to particular behaviors, characteristics and perceived accomplishments or deficits – "Oh you're wonderful. That's the best left-hook I've ever seen from a two-year old. Hit me again." With pre-verbal infants, the same distortion is delivered and received energetically when a caretaker is determined that the baby should feel a certain way. In both cases the responses of the adult are in excess of the child's internal experiences – a clear lack of attunement. While the child's overt behavior may seem to be responsive, the authentic Self is effectively overridden and the child is left to wonder where the truth lies. In terms of breathing room heavy over-mirroring is likely to generate enduring feelings of inundation.

At the other end of the continuum, 'under-mirroring' occurs when the parent or caregiver offers very few reflective responses, is not energetically 'present', or tends to respond significantly below the child's level of emotional intensity – " So your teacher gave you a gold star for arithmetic … that's nice dear. Now run along and play." With this type of mis-attunement, the mirror presented to the fledgling Self is lacking in clarity and form, leaving the child feeling empty, incomplete, insignificant and invisible. The underlying fear is abandonment.

In some cases these two parenting styles are combined to create a parenting strategy I call 'selective mirroring. This applies when attention is given to a child's 'desirable' expressions and attributes, while those considered unacceptable are ignored. In effect the mirror reflects only those aspects of the Self the parents wish to see – "That was such a nice smile you gave Uncle George after you stabbed his budgie with my knitting needle. You're such a happy boy." Joking aside in my personal and professional experience this type of mirroring is particularly common. In most cases it is laden with the conscious or unconscious agenda of well-meaning parents. Unfortunately it is also a prescription advocated by many professionals and many popular parent-training manuals. It's called 'focusing on the positive" or 'positive reinforcement.' Because of its pragmatic appeal, the injurious nature of selective mirroring is often unseen or denied. One of the most unfortunate outcomes is that the wonderful excitations, images and fantasies of childhood are systematically denied expression and prematurely extinguished, later replaced by flattened out adult versions of reality. In the longer term, children who are mirrored selectively usually end up with a Self divided between 'good' and 'bad'. Believing their acceptability to be highly conditional, they struggle to exhibit the former while concealing the latter – even from themselves. As the judgments of others become internalized, the repressed 'badness' is manifested through pervasive feelings of dissatisfaction, self-doubt and, above all, guilt. At the deepest level, these children are caught between fears of both abandonment and inundation and their attempts to move away from one only brings them closer to the other.

'Critical mirroring' is a more obvious form of mis-attunement and its effects more readily apparent. In this case, the authentic experiences of the child are constantly interrupted by negative 'introjects' of the parent – "Wipe that smile off your face, anybody can tie a shoe-lace. Just look, your boots are filthy." On the inside, feelings are not only discounted but also 'wronged'. On the outside behaviors are tagged as being undesirable, insufficient or plainly unacceptable. Children who look into this mirror, particular during infancy, will question their own rightness and have great difficulty in coming to see themselves as competent and worthwhile human beings. If the critical mirroring is intensive, their underlying fear will be one of inundation. On the other hand, if they are confronted by distant and generalized negativity they are likely to end up feeling rejected and abandoned.

For the most part, parent-child mirroring difficulties arise when the adult lacks a secure and integrated sense of

Self. This is particularly evident where a parent projects his or her own experience onto the child as a form of self-indulgence. Referred to as 'narcissistic mirroring, glimpses of the child's interior world are used as opportunities to bring substance to the adult's own tenuous and incomplete Self. My Aunt Rachel was brilliant at this. She would always ask me about my day at school, but as soon as I offered the first tidbit of information, she would launch out into an endless procession of stories about her own schooldays. Being a good boy, I would sit there pretending to listen and cursing myself for having been sucked in again. In effect, narcissistic mirroring is a smash and grab raid in which the invader breaks through the relational boundary to take over and dismiss the experiences of another. In the extreme case, the child is unable to establish a separate boundary and becomes absorbed into a confused state of merger with the parent. This tragic state of affairs, sometimes referred to as a 'solipsistic' relationship, creates a level of inundation in which the child is denied the most fundamental of all development needs – the assurance of his or her existence as a separate human being.

Establishing a clear and distinctive sense of Self is also a problem for children who receive inconsistent, distorted, or 'psychotic mirroring'. In each case recipients are presented with energetic and verbal feedback that is erratic, blurred, or fragmented – "Yes, I know you're feeling happy and that's good. Sometimes you're bad and that's not good is it? Perhaps it's good to be bad sometimes. Or perhaps you'd rather be sad." Inconsistency creates uncertainty, ambiguity and confusion, undermining the needs of the Self for clarity, coherence and continuity. Distorted mirroring can be more serious; twisting images into strange configurations like those we pay to laugh at in Amusement Parks. In rare cases, a child may be exposed to mirroring that is so inconsistent and distorted that even the fragments cannot be pieced together into any recognizable image. In the extreme these 'psychotic' mirroring forms create internal chaos and cognitive dissociation to the point where the child is unable to operate within the consensus of everyday reality. During my years working in residential treatment programs, I came across several children who had this kind of history and were assumed to be suffering from some form of psychotic disorder. Their pain was not the product of a diseased mind. The only thing wrong in their heads was that their brains struggled to make connections from the only information they had been given. The underlying problem was that these hopelessly lost Souls had never been granted the opportunity to establish a coherent sense of Self through their relationships with others and their dealings with the 'real' world.

ACCURATE MIRRORING

As an aspect of energetic and empathic attunement, accurate mirroring can never be considered an exact science. The above examples illustrate particular forms that may be injurious to the emerging Self of the child, but elements of such mis-attunements can be identified in all parent-child relationships. For the first three years of my own life, I was under-mirrored by a distracted mother and selectively mirrored by a very determined paternal grandmother. With my father absent for much of that time, I had no available mirror to reflect my maleness. In my family and culture, feelings were rarely discussed and emotions tightly held. Yet overall, there was enough there for me to feel wanted and loved.

The energetic attunement between a mother and her infant lays the foundation for the development of empathy - or empathic attunement.

Taken together my mirrors reflected constant images of a 'normal' and cared for little boy, even if my inner world was not generally seen and heard on the outside. Fortunately my father returned to the family as a full-time member when I was four, just when I most needed to see myself through the eyes of a loving male. I was well into my thirties before I got around to doing the personal work that made it possible for me to understand, share and let go of what that little boy had been hanging on to. At that point I knew enough to choose my mirrors very carefully.

In its purest form, accurate mirroring begins when a mother is able to communicate her warmth, love and acceptance, confirming her infant as a separate and unique human being. This is accomplished not so much through her actions as through her energetic presence. If she is distracted, out of touch with her own feelings or fearful, the communication will be proportionately compromised. If her own mirroring history is seriously flawed, her natural ability to sense and reflect the child's feelings will be diminished. And if her own sense of Self is incomplete and 'needy', she will be unable to accurately reflect her infant's separateness.

The energetic attunement between a mother and her infant lays the foundation for the development of empathy - or empathic attunement. A child who feels seen and heard in the primary relationship remains open to the experience of Self and Other and will bring this awareness into subsequent relationships. With the development of perceptual and cognitive abilities, this information becomes increasingly abstract and complex but the essential foundation of unmediated energetic contact remains intact.

In its most developed form, the ability to empathetically and accurately reflect the experiences of another person combines a number of essential ingredients.

- First and foremost, it requires a secure Self that is fully present and contained within its own boundary. Any confusion about where one person ends and the other begins will blur the images and contaminate the integrity of the mirror.

- The person offering the mirror must be open to his or her authentic feelings and thoughts, taking full ownership for these creations. There must be genuine curiosity and focused attention upon the experience of the other. Without this, the connection will be weak, and the mirroring responses will miss their target.

As a cognitive act between adults, the ability to place oneself in the position of another and look back through that person's eyes is an incredibly complex process. Often referred to 'role-taking', or 'perspective taking', this involves taking in masses of sensory information and drawing upon previous learning to create educated testable assumptions and hypotheses.

At the core, it is still the energetic quality of the connection that provides the channel for affective and verbal responses. Even when mirroring an adult, the words and gestures will always be secondary to the information transmitted and received energetically. If you question this, try having someone repeat your words in rote fashion and notice how it feels.

Above all, accurate mirroring demands that there be no agenda other than the desire to respond authentically to the experience of an Other. Any attempt to influence that experience or impose some external interpretation, consciously or unconsciously, transforms mirroring into manipulation.

The obvious implication is that anybody who enters into a relationship with a child or young person should be able to provide a responsive and accurate mirror. If you wish to offer this powerful developmental service, I suggest you begin by checking out your own early mirroring history. If you look carefully you will discover many deficiencies and biases that might be unwittingly passed on to others. As always, awareness is not enough. Unless you take remedial action, the gaps will always be there and however much you might try to contain the distortions they will find expression in one form or another. The solution is simple – find another person who is prepared to offer you a mirror. This should be a person who possesses a solid sense of Self and is willing to sit down and simply reflect whatever you wish to share about your world on the inside. Unfortunately such folks are few and far between, and you may be tempted to pay a professional for the experience. But be careful; most therapists have their own agenda and you may find yourself drawn into their version of treatment before the first session is over.

My preferred alternative is to choose a person with whom you already have a meaningful relationship and invite them to participate in an exercise we call "exchanging mirrors". This involves taking turns to practice mirroring while the other uses breathing as means of contacting and expressing the immediate responses of the authentic Self. You may not find yourself looking into an accurate mirror in the first few sessions, but with continued practice and constant feedback the images will become increasingly clear and illuminating. As an added bonus, you will also begin to see how your own gaps, biases and agendas get in the way of your own ability to mirror an Other. We have found this exercise particularly useful in our work with couples. In many cases, they report seeing each other 'for the first time' after many years of false assumptions, projections and illusions. Anyone interested in experimenting with this method will find a more detailed overview at the end of this book (see appendix B). Meanwhile the good news is that it's never too late to be accurately mirrored, whatever your age or developmental history.

THE SCIENCE OF MIRRORING

For those who like to have the hard-core scientific evidence, neuroscientist Marco Iacoboni takes it straight out of the laboratory in his book *Mirroring People* published in 2008. With great enthusiasm he talks about the discovery of "smart cells" that enable our brain to understand others. Here he finds the 'seeds' of empathy and social cognition, and uncovers the neural pathways that enable us to get inside another person's head. It makes for interesting reading, but once again, it seems to me like another example of science catching up with what we already know. Of course the fundamental question is whether we do these things because our brains are programmed in this way, or whether we make use of, or even create, the neural systems that enable us to experience and express our humanity with each other? The choice is yours – or is it?

MESSAGES WITHOUT WORDS

Returning to the energetic connection between a mother and her pre-verbal infant, I have already suggested that the state of communion contains vital information for the receptive Self of the child. The message "I love you," for example, is a powerful energetic assurance that the bond is strong, and the infant can bask securely in the warmth of mother's affection. Over time this message becomes incorporated into the basic structure of the emerging Self as an enduring statement or attribution – "I am lovable." At some point along the developmental pathway, this becomes translated into the relational statement – "I am lovable, and so are you." In other words what the infant received and internalized can now be passed on to others, with or without reciprocity. I believe it's impossible to over emphasize the importance of this foundational learning, but above all I want to stress that it occurs pre-verbally, is facilitated energetically and contained somatically – as a felt sense in the body.

Important as the "I love you" message might be, there are many others that may be consciously or unconsciously conveyed by a parent, each in its own way becoming incorporated into the deep structures of the infant Self. In their book *The Intimate Couple*, Jack Lee Rosenberg and Beverly Kitaen-Morse offer a list of what they call "Good Mother" and "Good Father" messages. These categories are used only to distinguish the earliest messages from those that tend to become more significant as the child grows older. In fact any message can come from either parent and both should convey all messages. At one level, these are endorsements that every child would benefit from receiving from the outset. Fundamentally, they are the affirmations from which a child is able to develop an integrated, worthwhile and expressive Self. While I have stressed the importance of energetic communication, particularly during the pre-verbal period, these affirmations are imparted through many channels. In the words of Rosenberg and Kitaen-Morse, "the good parent messages are supported by words and deeds but, without the full energetic quality that comes from openness, authenticity, and presence in the givers, the messages are empty" (p.26).

As you read the statements listed below, you may wish to consider the implications of each one from the perspective of a child preparing for life's uncertainties. Obviously they are not scientifically verifiable and you may find yourself wanting to add to the list. But after working with these messages personally and professionally for many years, I feel no need to create additions. Like so much of Rosenberg's work, they are founded upon well-established psychological principles, blended with remarkable insight and drawn from many years of clinical experience. Using my own test of scientific-subjectivity, I have no hesitation in awarding my personal seal of validity to the following:

GOOD MOTHER MESSAGES

1. *I love you*
2. *I want you*
3. *You are special to me*
4. *I see you and I hear you*
5. *It's not what you do but who you are that I love*
6. *I love you, and I give you permission to be different from me*
7. *I'll take care of you*
8. *I'll be there for you; I will be there even when you die*
9. *You don't have to be alone anymore*
10. *You can trust me*
11. *You can trust your inner voice*
12. *Sometimes I will tell you "no," and that's because I love you*
13. *You don't have to be afraid anymore*
14. *My love will make you well*
15. *I welcome and cherish your love*

GOOD FATHER MESSAGES

1. *I can set limits, and I am willing to enforce them*
2. *If you fall down, I will pick you up*
3. *I am proud of you*
4. *I have confidence in you; I am sure you will succeed*
5. *I give you permission to be the same as I, to be more, or less*
6. *You are beautiful (handsome)*
7. *I give you permission to love and enjoy your erotic sexuality with a partner of your choice and not lose me.*

For anyone tempted to use these statements as a check-list for evaluating his or her own parenting performance, the creators are quick to point out that nobody has ever received all the messages completely and perfectly. Whatever deficiencies are identified (and there could be many) the vast majority of parents send their children off with a package that will sustain them through the early stages of life's adventure. The more children receive and internalize these messages, however, the more they will set out with a belief in themselves and confidence in their ability to manage their own lives in their own way. Even more to the point, they will have a firm foundation for the on going development of the Self through the creation of meaningful and mutually satisfying relationships.

It is important to understand that the good parent messages are received and internalized in early childhood. As the child begins to formulate a cognitive view of Self – a self-concept if you like – the information becomes assimilated into an internal belief system that filters and mediates the incoming messages. Once this is established, external feedback that is disturbing or contrary to the internal perspective is systematically modified or rejected in the service of maintaining a solid and coherent self-concept – a process which psychologists refer to as 'avoiding cognitive dissonance.' Yet the need for these self-assurances does not diminish, and the chances are the child will move into adulthood still seeking the affirmations that were not available at the time when the self-system was open and receptive. Since others can never provide such satisfaction - not even the parents at this age - this fruitless search for assurance can profoundly affect the person's ability to create satisfying and lasting relationships. This unhappy state of affairs can only be resolved when he or she realizes that the missing messages can only come from the inside through self-validation, or more descriptively, through 'self-parenting.'

To reiterate a familiar theme, adults cannot offer a good parent message they never received – either from their parents or through their own self-validation. As always the task of identifying the missing pieces begins with awareness, and the remedial work is accomplished through self-directed effort. Personally I have found working with these messages to be an incredibly rewarding exercise for anyone who wishes to move beyond his or her own early developmental interruptions and injuries. The internal dialogue opens up a channel of communication between the mind and the Self that enables the person to modify old patterns of thinking, feeling and behaving, from the inside out. This in turn, opens up new opportunities for the Self to become an active creator of relationships, rather than a dissatisfied and dependent accomplice. The ability to inform, nurture and endorse one's own Self makes it possible for a parent to offer those messages that would otherwise be missing and prevent the deficiencies from being passed on to the next generation. A parent who has done this work possesses a gift that would be priceless to any child fortunate enough to stand and gaze into such a consistent, integrated and reliable mirror.

> *This ... opens up new opportunities for the Self to become an active creator of relationships, rather than a dissatisfied and dependent accomplice.*

If you're seriously interested in working with the good parent messages, you could do no better than follow the procedures suggested by Rosenberg and Kitaen-Morse. Begin by reading through the good mother messages. After two or three minutes, write down those you can remember and then go back to the original list. Repeat this each day for two or three days, paying particular attention to those you keep forgetting. The chances are that these will be the messages you didn't receive or are still seeking. As you read each statement, take a deep breath and you will notice that each message feels different. In the words of Rosenberg and Kitaen-Morse: "Each message elicits a distinct body experience that can be identified in a different part of your body. 'I love you' feels different from 'I want you' or 'you are special to me' and so on." (p.27 B)

Remember it isn't so much the words themselves that matter, but the energetic or somatic experiences associated with each statement. This applies to your responses as well as to ways you decide to "give" yourself a particular message. Simply repeating the words without the authentic and caring feelings, will never take the message to its intended recipient – the core Self. You may wish to write the messages down as you convey them. Alternatively you may wish to sing them, paint them, or create a verse around them – whatever it takes to communicate with the deeper levels of the Self. You may also decide to direct them to those aspects of your Self that seem to need them the most. There is no single prescription that fits for all. Your sense of Self is like no other, and the dialogue you create will need to reflect that uniqueness. So sit back, relax, and have a wonderful journey into wholeness. Meanwhile, I will return to my own project.

The Basic Fault

Before leaving the lessons of early childhood I want to go back even further, to that time and place when mother first moved out of sync with our most primary needs, bringing about our earliest confrontations with the Nemo. In his book, *The Basic Fault*, published in 1968, psychiatrist Michael Balint argues that, since this is a universal feature of the human condition, we all must find ways to deal with the fears that arise when our sense of connection to the world is unexpectedly interrupted. His use of the term 'fault' has two interrelated meanings or dimensions. One is a geological metaphor and relates to the structural displacements that occur within the matrix of our relational life. The other is more psychological and refers to the body-feeling of emptiness that surface at times when the continuity of our lives appears to be threatened. The underlying sense is that something is wrong, something is missing, and we struggle to make sense of our condition. More often than not, the answer that follows is one with which we are only too familiar – a recurring response learned early in childhood and now entrenched in both body and mind. It may take the form of self-derogation – "I am useless," "I am a sinner," "I am unlovable." Or it might be directed at the world in general – "Nobody cares," "I'm all alone," "Nobody can be trusted." Whatever the particular belief and regardless of the available evidence, the same response of finding fault with Self, Other, or the world in general, continues to repeat itself. Using a computer analogy it's like a default position that's prompted when the on-going system fails or is in some way interrupted. As most of us know only too well, when the software is by-passed and the hard drive takes over, the repetitive responses are virtually impossible to modify or eradicate. This means that any attempts to change the particular words, attitudes and beliefs are pointless. These are not the basic faults, only the machinations of the mind's software. We may not be able to remove the source of the problem, but we may discover ways to recognize it when it appears and intervene to reduce its influence on our lives. Allow me to offer a personal example that might help to put some flesh on Balint's conceptual bones.

Sometimes when my immediate ambitions are thwarted, I'm still inclined to deny my own volition and attribute my discontent to forces beyond my control. I might even look heavenward and demand divine intervention or at least, accountability. In most cases I catch myself quickly and find some amusement in my stupidity. But there are odd times when I slip through the restraints of rationality and find myself sinking into a self-indulgent quagmire. This could be prompted by something as simple as trying to fix a hinge on the door of a kitchen cabinet. Rather than acknowledge my lack of presence, commitment and skill, I choose to vent my frustration upon a screwdriver with its own perverse agenda, or a screw that insists on falling out of its hole and onto the floor every time I have everything nicely lined up. I have been known to punish such recalcitrant hardware unmercifully.

Climbing back onto the chair for the third time and gripping the base of the cabinet for support, that laminated lay-about uses my momentary dependency as an excuse to part company with the wall. Seizing the opportunity to wreak revenge on the backside that has committed a thousand insults, the chair decides to keel over and send me crashing to the deck. Right on cue my distraught partner makes her entrance. But her concern is not for my well being. Oh no, the tears in her eyes are for the bone china dinner service I neglected to remove from the now deceased cabinet before commencing operations. It's just another part of a cold-blooded conspiracy. If she hadn't stored her precious platters in that pig of a cupboard, nagged on about the damned hinge and stubbornly refused to call in 'Fred the Fixer,' I wouldn't be dragging myself off the kitchen floor surrounded by vicious shards of hand-painted debris. My rage is escalating and turning in her direction. It's time for she and I to create distance, at least until the storm subsides. I head for the shelter of my office.

Like a man hanging over a cliff, all the frenetic gestures, screaming and scrambling creates only a brief respite from the cruel course of destiny. Sitting with my elbows on the desk and my head in my hands I know I'm slipping, but I fight on. It isn't my fault. I didn't want to mess with that cupboard in the first place. I hate that fucking cupboard. The fury begins to abate, turning into a sickly sadness. Why can't I be recognized for the things I can do and not just condemned for the things I can't? I'm tiring now; my mind is weary, my body drained of substance. You've never been good at the stuff men are supposed to do. You were a laughing stock in woodwork. Even your own father gave up on you – remember the incident with the gas can? I continue my descent. Just face it; you're not very good at being a man at all. It's just a façade... a pathetic pretence... you're a phony man... an imposter hiding the shame of your incompetence. I'm dissolving into my belly, the echoes of my laments fading into nowhere. I'm in the hole, the dark place were even the boldest shadows lose their form. No more words, no more thoughts - only the nauseating silence. Now, from somewhere deep within the blackness I hear the distant cries of a child. I try to close my ears but this pitiful voice is not from the outside – Is anybody there? I'm all alone down here. Give me another chance. I'll do whatever you say. Please help me.

What we need to understand is that, at its core, the basic fault is a body-feeling that has its origins long before we had thoughts and words to account for our experiences. As adults we need to recognize how this confrontation with our most basic fears continues to interfere with our lives by disrupting our sense of certainty, constancy and continuity. Only then are we able to focus our attention on changing that which is possible – our cognitive and behavioral responses. This is where Jack Lee Rosenberg steps back into the picture. In his unpublished notes, he suggests the following:

1. To bring your basic fault to awareness, write the feeling that you consistently have about yourself when you are 'off,' (e.g.) "I'm not good enough, I'm bad, I've done something wrong, I'm all alone. No one in my life is worthy of trust.

2. Identify the feeling in your body that shows up when you feel this theme. Link up the above psychological narrative with the body-feeling.

3. Memorize this mantra: That's the way any little (boy or girl) would feel who had a mother who didn't receive (constancy, physical affection etc) and therefore couldn't give it.

4. Repeat this sentence each time the thought or body message arises into your awareness. To release its power over us, the basic fault must be identified as defining the past, not the present.

This may sound like a superficial solution to a very profound problem but the brilliance of Rosenberg is in his ability to identify the simple that lies beyond the complex. This you will discover for yourself if you take the time to read his seminal text *Body, Self and Soul*. In this work, he takes the most sophisticated forms of psychotherapy including psychoanalysis, and distills them into a form that makes 'simple' intuitive sense to anyone who 'simply' wishes to understand.

The Case of a Little Girl Who Stayed Inside

Throughout this chapter I have attempted to identify some of the primary issues that arise from our earliest relational experiences. Looking back I realize I have covered a lot of territory, using many abstract thoughts and concepts to explicate and support my position. Throughout it all, my primary objective has been to identify those aspects of early childhood that shape our lives, specifically those factors that serve to promote or inhibit our development as self-directed and self-responsible human beings. I have tried to pay particular attention to the task of parenting, keeping in mind the implications for anyone fortunate enough to be involved in the lives of children. Before concluding this section I would like to ground some of these abstractions within the history of a twelve year old girl I met a long time ago – I'll call her Laura. Please know from the outset that this is not your run-of-the-mill family narrative. I have selected this story because it dramatically exemplifies so many of the relational factors involved in early development.

I first heard about Laura through a telephone call from a consulting psychiatrist in Toronto. Apparently Laura was referred to him at the insistence of a school principal who wanted to know why this otherwise exemplary student never spoke in class, and made no attempt to make contact with the other students. Psychological testing presented the profile of a twelve-year old girl with above average intelligence, age-appropriate cognitive development and significantly limited social awareness. Still, there was nothing that might account for her total lack of communication in and around the school. The records from previous schools generally reported her to be a "good student," although some references were made to her "quietness" or "shyness" in the classroom and one teacher expressed concern about her "lack of friends."

When the psychiatrist agreed to see her for an assessment, Laura made no eye contact and said nothing even when the questions were simple and direct. Her only shift in affect was the faintest hint of a smile when he showed her a book of animal cartoons. In a second follow-up session, he attempted to engage her non-verbally through a series of interactive games, but there was no interaction – no contact.

With his standard diagnostic methods seemingly ineffective, the psychiatrist invited the parents and two older sons to his office in the hope of finding some clues somewhere within the dynamics of the family. Although they all insisted that Laura was "not like this at home," nobody made any effort to draw her into the discussion.

From this observation alone, the psychiatrist concluded that something was going on in the family that should be investigated. His recommendation was that Laura be temporarily removed from the home for individual assessment and treatment and the family, including Laura involved in on going family therapy. I agreed, and accepted the referral on the understanding that the family would be prepared to travel a considerable distance to attend the family sessions.

When I first saw Laura, she was standing with her parents in the foyer of the girl's 'cottage.' Her head was bowed so I couldn't see her face, but her overall appearance was not what you might expect of a 12 year old girl being admitted to a residential treatment centre. She was wearing a short white coat over a blue cotton dress with matching blue patent leather shoes. Her arms were wrapped around a heavily embroidered handbag, clasped tightly to her stomach. With her head angled forward, the long curls of her blonde hair fell across her cheeks, forming a veil that made the contours of her face even more inaccessible. Yet what was really striking about the drooping figure standing between two very upright parents was that everything about her was immaculate. Even her stance could have been carefully sculpted to create the perfect image of dejection, framed by pillars of strength and resolve on either side. Taken together they could have been a parody on some version of a Normal Rockwell creation.

Throughout the hour-long admission meeting that involved myself, the parents, and two members of the child and youth care team, Laura sat motionless on her chair in the circle. She would present only the top of her head to the gathering. Meanwhile, everybody else went on with the matters at hand as if she wasn't there. There were brief moments when I sensed she really was 'there' only to disappear again. I also noticed that mother seemed to glance across at her daughter at precisely those moments. It was all speculation on my part, but sufficient to arouse my curiosity about the relationship between this elusive young girl in the blue dress and her upright mother.

When the meeting was over we left Laura and her parents to exchange their parting words, and though I was tempted to eavesdrop – strictly for assessment purposes of course - I made my way back to my office for my next appointment. An hour or so later as I was preparing for the evening group therapy session, one of the residential staff came to tell me that Laura was still sitting in the meeting room refusing to budge. Sure enough, I found her just as we had left her. She made no response to my arrival, my greeting or my announcement that it was time for her to settle into her room. On my way out of the residence, I left instructions that she should be left exactly where she was, but respond to her positively if she made any statement or request.

It was late in the evening when I checked back, only to discover that nothing had changed. She was still sitting in the chair, her posture drooped and her chin now on her chest. A number of the other residents had visited and invited her to join in the evening's activities but to no avail. Now they were ignoring her. Before going home, I scribbled my instructions into the communication book; "Look in on Laura every five minutes and ask if there's anything she needs. If no response, leave. If she makes any request, respond positively and immediately call me at home." Before going to bed I telephoned the residence – still no change.

On my arrival the following morning, both staff and residents confronted me. All expressed their concern about the solitary figure in the meeting room. As I approached the door, I was greeted by the sickly stench of stale urine. Following my instructions to the letter, the night staff had offered to take her to the bathroom, but since she made no response, they had taken no action. Now the other girls were in on the act, holding their noses and expressing their disgust as they walked by. Laura was still in the same place, but she was no longer the immaculate girl who had stood in the foyer the day before. She was slumped forward; her hair was greasy and bedraggled; the collar of her white coat was now pulled up over her ears; and her blue cotton dress clung tightly around her knees. I immediately decided not to push the matter any further and asked a female counselor to escort her to the bathroom, make sure she was appropriately cleansed, and then deposit her in room. As I sat in my office ruminating over this decision, one of the male night counselors stuck his head in the door to offer an insightful and astute observation. "Isn't it interesting," he said. "One little girl can capture everybody's concern and attention by doing absolutely nothing." "It certainly is," I replied. "But I wonder what would happen in the long run if we all remained firm and did absolutely nothing in return." "Well I'm out of here," he said. "Have a good day." "Oh, thanks," I said.

Much as I would enjoy telling you about our subsequent work with Laura, this isn't the purpose of the exercise. My project is to apply the ideas outlined earlier in this chapter to explain how this unhappy little girl ended up in a residential treatment centre. In case you feel set up or ripped-off by this, I'll add a synopsis of our work later. Meanwhile let me begin by outlining the circumstances that brought Laura into the world.

Her parents met as students at a religious college in Ontario. Bart was in his final year and preparing to become a minister; Faye was in only her second semester, seeking to find some role for herself, as a woman, within a church community. Bart was a "good man," charismatic, ambitious and obviously "going places." When Faye listened to him preach, it "sounded like a voice from

Heaven … I could see the light around him." To serve him would be to serve God. To Bart, Faye seemed like the perfect companion. She was a "good woman," gentle, thoughtful and kind. And since his God was her God, she would be a wonderful support for his career and make a fine mother for his children. And so it came to pass – or so it seemed.

For the first ten years of their marriage, Bart and Faye presented themselves as the quintessential committed, caring, Christian couple. They had two apple-cheeked children, both boys, and Bart's career, while not spectacular, gave them a solid and respected place in the local community. Even so, beneath the ornate carvings and velvet trimmings of the marital pulpit, a Specter of darkness lurked ominously in the vaults. Bart was having an affair. This wasn't a passing fancy, the kind of thing married men sometimes do; this was another woman, from another town. Faye was torn apart when she discovered her husband's betrayal, but the trauma was never brought into the light. It was a secret they kept from each other, as well as the outside world. The door to the vaults was locked and sealed.

Faye blamed herself. She had failed as a wife, just as she had failed as a daughter. It was her birth that brought about the death of her mother and it was her carnal transgression with a distant cousin that had sent her father into a fit of rage, calling upon the wrath of God to punish his 'incestuous' daughter. It was she who had committed unspeakable acts. She was the sinner who must search for peace through atonement and hopefully, forgiveness. This is why she went into the seminary and why she chose to serve God through His agent, Bart. He was the goodness that would serve to ameliorate her badness. Now she was alone again, with nothing between her and the eternal voice of judgment.

For her part she had tried to be perfect in every way as a wife, a mother and a devoted servant of the Church. Her husband's growing ministry and her two well-mannered boys were living testimony to her commitment. Clearly, it wasn't enough and the other woman had come along to deliver the message that her atonement was not complete. Her husband had broken his vows and could no longer speak to the Almighty on her behalf. Within a few years, her boys would be off to college and she would be destined to live out her life as a solitary sinner. There could be no more children. When their younger son was born after a tenuous pregnancy, her doctor had recommended a complete hysterectomy but she declined, believing that God was the sole guardian of her womb. She agreed with Bart that they should 'take all necessary precautions,' while continuing to pray for a miracle that would allow her one more child, a daughter who would retrieve the lost innocence of her own childhood and put a smile on the face of the Lord. Satisfying herself that it would have to be His decision, she wrapped her diaphragm in a Kleenex and tucked it away in her bedroom drawer. After another shaky pregnancy and traumatic delivery, Laura arrived eleven months later.

To say she was born into a powerful parental agenda would be an obvious understatement. Whatever problems were waiting to surface, they would not arise from any deficiency in the maternal bond. Faye's compelling need for her daughter ensured that mother would 'be there,' savoring every moment of connection and making sure than even the most fleeting infantile needs were immediately identified and satisfied. In this sense energetic attunement was not a problem either; in fact Faye became so tuned-in to her daughter's state of being that she was able to anticipate the baby's desires and discomforts before they actually occurred. This gave her great pleasure and she spent countless hours challenging her insight and practicing her skills. From the outside she was the exemplary mother and even Bart, who had campaigned strongly for an abortion, openly acknowledged that his wife was everything a mother should be. He watched over her with gentle eyes, spoke proudly of her devotion in his sermons and proclaimed Laura to be a 'little angel sent from Heaven.' With the attention of the congregation upon the family, his out-of-town 'visitations' became too risky and he made arrangements to relocate the other woman and his other child. Relieved of what had become an obligation, he had his own reasons for thanking baby Laura. Her large brown eyes and gentle whimpers had summoned him back to his wife's side and reunited their family. It was meant to be.

The problem of course, was 'breathing room' (see page 218) and that problem was severe. Faye projected everything good about herself onto her baby and took everything innocent in return. Who could ever deny that beautiful Laura was a gift from God, the confirmation of His love, the healer of her husband's betrayal and above all, the key to her own reconciliation with the Divine? But this was all in Faye's mind. From beneath, the hollow cries of the deeply flawed and incomplete Self of a sinner percolated through even the slightest fracture in their union, and the misery would return. So she held on tight, vigilant, anticipating possible breaches and moving quickly to seal the inevitable gaps.

The mirror she offered contained only her own fragmented and tormented image, along with her desperate need to be loved without conditions or judgments. She reflected only what she wanted to see, ignoring or smothering anything that might keep them apart. There were photographs everywhere – Laura in mother's arms wearing her pink dress and lace booties; Laura and mother together on the front lawn, on the living room sofa, in the bathtub, at the christening; and everybody smiled. Nobody asked why there were no pictures of Laura on her own.

Yet always there were fears, vague and fleeting at first but gradually closing in as the baby became a toddler, and the toddler began to utter her first words. Faye knew exactly what she wanted her daughter to say, but there were slippages - unacceptable demands and inappropriate revelations, violations of their wordless contract blurted out in front of strangers. When Laura was silent and smiling, Faye would draw her close and kiss her cheek and the onlookers would beam. Later they would eat cake, just the two of them and talk to Teddy in their pink-petal playroom. If Laura misbehaved with her words, the hand that drew her close gripped tightly, the smile was rigid and the kiss cold. Faye always waited until they were together in the 'quiet room' before any words were allowed to pass between them. "We were naughty in Mrs. Robson's shop this afternoon weren't we? When we're naughty like that, Teddy doesn't want to talk to us and Daddy doesn't love us. Now we must be very good when Daddy takes us to market tomorrow. We want Daddy to love us because we love Daddy. Then we'll come home and tell Teddy all about it."

For Faye, the anticipation of her daughter going to school was unbearable. She had set her heart on a program of home schooling, but Bart would have none of it. In desperation she offered her services as a teacher's aide, but the principal would give no assurance she would be assigned to Laura's class. She insisted on knowing who the teacher would be and went to see her. But Miss Fletcher was equally non-committal, obviously wanting to keep Laura to herself. So Faye convinced her husband to pay for their daughter to attend a private school. Here she was given permission to 'drop in' whenever she had the time or the inclination. It wasn't an ideal arrangement but Faye had no choice other than to make the best of it. And she did.

I have no reason to dwell on Laura's story any further. Hopefully you will already have the picture of a lost little girl with an overwhelming and impossible task to perform. Her refusal to speak in public was the learned response of a Self that was denied definition, expression, and individuation. In and of itself, her reticence was not 'the problem' but it was a key factor in stifling the Self and maintaining the solipsistic relationship between mother and child.

If you believe Faye was the sole creator of Laura's diminished life, she may have agreed with you; she was, after all, a self-denounced sinner responsible for the anguish of others and the wrath of the Almighty. If you were to look carefully into the relational patterns of her family, however, you would see that she too was robbed of her childhood and carried her crosses with as much strength and dignity as she could muster. You may also be tempted to overlook the role of Bart in all of this. Preoccupied by his ministerial ambitions, he offered very little support and understanding for his struggling wife and turned his back on Laura's plight. He was cold and distant from his children, while parading the glossy tableau of his family before his gullible flock. Again, his own family history reveals the struggles of a young lad abandoned by his mother and driven by the constant demands of bible-thumping father.

I'm not pointing this out to make excuses or let anybody off the hook. In the final analysis, we are all responsible for the choices we make in dealing with the legacies of childhood, but this simple assertion should never be used as substitute for empathy and understanding. We are all human beings on our own developmental pathway and there's no way that one person's life can be understood or evaluated through the moralistic judgments of another. Our own injuries and challenges may seem less severe than Laura's, but perhaps that's only because they are less obvious. If we are to retain our privileged place on this planet, the time has come for us to look beyond the simplistic and superficial and embrace the spirituality of our wholeness. As individuals we are not good or bad. Nor are we some combination of the two. In the eyes of the universal Mother, we are all seeking to reclaim the truth of our connectedness.

Before ending this chapter, I want to honor my commitment to provide you with a brief overview of our work with Laura at the Centre. Since this book is not about 'treatment' or 'therapy, I will skim over the details and focus on the elements and highlights I consider to be significant.

From the day of her admission we realized nothing of significance would happen until we could establish some kind of personal contact with Laura. Having explored many ways to achieve this, including long silent marathons, combined with simple everyday routines and courtesies, we fell back on the old principle that much of what has been learned can be unlearned. Since her reticence was a response to mother's selective mirroring and rewarding, we decided to use the same approach in reverse – mirroring her independence and rewarding any expressive behaviors. In other words, we set out with a highly structured program of behavior modification. Given what I have said before about manipulating a child's behavior through external contingencies and controls this may surprise you, but what needs to be recognized is that the behaviors we were attempting to 'elicit' were seen as a means to an end, and not an end in themselves.

In general, we were looking for behaviors that indicated any responsiveness to others. Ideally we hoped to establish face-to-face or even eye contact but we would need to build up to this through a process of successive approximations known in the trade as 'shaping.' First we had to find rewards that would elicit and strengthen, or 'reinforce,' these behaviors. In Laura's case the usual social rewards of approval and personal closeness were clearly ineffective. In fact they were more than likely to intensify her withdrawal. Knowing she was an avid stamp collector, and thanks to a staff member who offered to sacrifice his modest collection to the cause, we put together a workable supply of rewards. However contrived this might seem, and sparing you the details of the procedures, the fact is the program worked. Beginning with simple gestures, like reaching out to take a stamp from someone's hand, it was only a matter of days before Laura was nodding in response to questions and coming to the staff office unescorted. But she would always stand motionless in the doorway, her head characteristically bowed until the designated child and youth care worker was ready to take her and the box of stamps to the 'quiet room.'

The memory of looking directly into Laura's face for the first time will never be erased. She was sitting in my office with her usual slumped posture - head down, hands clasped and knees together. I was at my desk totally engrossed in a consultant's report, when some minor energetic shift prompted me to look up. There she was, her face fully exposed and her eyes seemingly directed toward something over my left shoulder. My first impression was that of a Japanese mannequin without the make up. Her skin was stretched tightly across her cheekbones, pulling her mouth into a fixed and lifeless smile. It was the strained cosmetic face of serenity that reveals absolutely nothing. I glanced over my shoulder and realized her attention was drawn to 'Cedrick,' my beloved porcelain Court Jester, who dangled his feet over the top of my bookshelf. Lifting out of my chair, I moved to position myself between Laura and Cedrick and for the briefest moment, her pale blue eyes seemed to be on me. If we made any contact at all it was gone in a flash, and I found myself staring into frozen hollows that held no sign of life and offered no reflection in return. She simply 'wasn't there,' and through those empty eyes, neither was I. The chill of my own aloneness spread from my belly to my bones and I began to tremble. In this fleeting encounter with eternity, this inscrutable little girl had brought me to the very edge. "This is Cedrick," I said, sitting him on my desk. "Do you like him?" Her head had dropped, but she managed to respond with the nod that no longer required a stamp. "Then come and see me in the morning and perhaps you can keep him for a while." She nodded again.

As I mentioned, it was not our intention to modify Laura's behavior and leave it at that. Our broader objective was to make contact and establish a relationship through which the locked-in Self might begin to move toward expression and freedom. For this purpose she was given her own exclusive child and youth care worker, a middle-aged woman who had been particularly successful during the early stages of the work. Whenever a stamp was delivered Cheryl would follow-up immediately with verbal feedback – a mirroring statement or an authentic expression of pleasure. Over time we noticed that Laura began to respond more to Cheryl than the anticipation of a stamp, and the feedback became more diverse and personal. There were times when Laura would make sounds, brief exhalations even the odd whisper, but despite her worker's encouragement, she steadfastly refused to transform these rudimentary vocalizations into actual words.

At this point I could sense Cheryl's frustration and how it was becoming increasingly difficult for her to maintain authentic positive feelings toward her speechless partner. Sitting in my office, gazing idly out of the window I happened to see Laura and four or five other girls playing around on the front lawn. I couldn't hear their voices so I began to watch their interaction patterns. I was struck by how popular Laura seemed to have become when I suddenly remembered the comments of the night worker who dropped into my office on that first morning. He saw something the rest of us were refusing to see or acknowledge – our dear Laura had everybody on the run. She had been singled out for 'special' treatment; people responded to her with warmth and gentle kindness. Staff and residents alike wanted to help, often anticipating her needs and trying to meet them through trial and error. Meanwhile she continued to withhold the one thing they all hoped for in return – a few words from those tightly sealed lips. Yet she kept their hopes alive with occasional hints of future possibilities - "Laura smiled at me today." "No kidding. Paul said she whispered something to him in the rec. room on Tuesday." "Really?… Wow."

With some dismay, I realized how my concern for Laura, along with my determination to make something happen, had distracted me from the obvious. On the one hand, we were responding with gentle sensitivity to a girl who had suffered enormous developmental damage. On the other, we were dealing with a very adept manipulator who was using her 'symptoms' to control everyone around her. If my mind had been open I might have seen this aspect as far back as the admission meeting, when Laura's subtle energetic shifts seemed to elicit mother's immediate attention and concern. In our in-service training programs, I always made a point of warning about the dangers of single-minded approaches and stressed the need to constantly step back and view the picture from different angles. Just like the old black and white drawing of the vase that can also be seen as two facial profiles, it's impossible to see a person's life from two distinct perspectives at the same time; you can only shift from one to the other. As professionals in the field we should have the ability to take multiple perspectives, albeit one at a time. Now I had managed to draw an entire team into my own myopia – a case of the blind leading the blind.

A few days later, after I had humbly confessed to my guilt and expressed my remorse at the team meeting, I walked past a clump of girls hanging around in the hallway. After throwing out a cheerless "Hi" to the group at large, I focused my attention on the drooping figure dangling on the periphery. "Oh Laura, I think you still have Cedrick in your room. Would you bring him back to my office please?" She turned away and began to shake her head. Usually I would have walked off but this time I decided to press my point. "I want to take him to my meeting with the little guys in Cottage Five tonight. Please have him back before dinner." Now she went into her familiar stance of resistance – body trembling, hands tightly clasped and head shaking from side-to-side. Rather than back off, I moved toward her and she reacted by shuffling into the middle of the group. "Laura," I said firmly, "this isn't a game. I want him back." As the girls closed ranks around her she made two rapid movements of the jaw and the others immediately burst into gasps of surprise, followed by elation and laughter. "What did she say?" I demanded to know, with little regard for the significance of the event. The other girls continued to laugh and giggle, preferring to give their attention to Laura rather than attend to my inquiry. "So, what did she say?" I asked again, with even more authority. Finally, a face rose from the excited huddle. "She told you to fuck off," said Margie with obvious satisfaction. This was greeted by another eruption of hilarity. "Not very appropriate for a minister's daughter," I remarked but in the madness of it all, my words were taken as irrelevant. If social approval provides powerful reinforcement for our behaviors, Laura received enough in that one incident to keep her cussing for a lifetime.

I'd like to tell you this was a carefully considered and timely intervention on my part, but the truth is I just wanted Cedrick back without having to be dragged through a maze of silent and senseless negotiations. I'd also like to report that, from this point on, our work with Laura was plain sailing. In actuality it was only the beginning; one significant step in building the relationship from which Laura might begin to take charge of her own life - from the inside out. For this she was in the residential program for over a year and would have remained longer had it not been for her father's transfer to a church in Oklahoma. Mother was receiving treatment for depression and both parents decided that it was time for their daughter to return to the family. Through detailed reports and lengthy telephone calls, I passed the work over to professionals in Tulsa and agreed to act as an external consultant. But my services were never called upon. Almost two years later, I received a call from a school psychologist in Austin, Texas. He was working with a girl called Laura who refused to speak and having read one of my reports, wondered if I had any suggestions to offer.

CHAPTER SIX

The Not-Too-Terrible Twos

If expressed affection and passive obedience are the measure of a 'good' child, then the period between eighteen months and three years can certainly be a challenge. Many parents will tell you this was a time when their kids behaved like trainee psychopaths, claiming exclusive ownership over everything in sight, demanding instant gratification, screaming for attention and not giving a tinker's toss for anybody else. All you have to do is spend a couple of hours in any shopping mall and you'll see exactly what they mean. How many times have you been tempted to pick up one of these little monsters by scruff and deposit him or her in the middle of the parking lot? Not me, of course – I'm a professional.

Can this be the same innocent soul that gazed into mother's eyes, seeking only to be cradled in the warmth of their communion? Is this the baby that cooed back at Daddy and laughed when Uncle Charlie pulled those stupid faces? Whatever became of the toddler who fell into Mommy's arms after that first ambulatory stumble across the living room floor? Before you answer, let me ask some similar questions from the other side of the fence. How do you respond to the sight of a parent shouting at, or even spanking, a young child for misbehaving in public? How many times have you watched a child being dragged down the aisle of a supermarket for attempted larceny at the candy counter? And what about the child sentenced to solitary confinement for snatching a ball from a younger brother or sister? Can these punishing enforcers be the same parents that once sat up most of the night just to watch their 'little treasure' sleep. Is this the same Momma who beamed at every burp? Whatever became of the Daddy who couldn't wait to get home from work just to hold a precious daughter in his arms?

Your answers to the above questions will, of course, depend upon the particular perspective you choose to take. If you begin with the assumption that each person possesses a unique essence, then you will see an underlying theme of continuity in every life. If you take the position from which each life is seen as a complex interaction among genetic, biological and social variables, then such continuity is a narrative constructed from the basic laws of nature. You may be tempted to follow in the footsteps of those who have attempted to combine these two perspectives within a single framework, but this is nothing more than a convenient sham. Unlike evolution and creationism, these are distinct and mutually exclusive positions that, through extrapolation grow further and further apart. If you are unsure where you stand in this matter, I suggest you begin by adopting one position or the other and use this as a constant point of reference for your observations and speculations. Whichever stance you take, my only hope is that you make your position clear and apply it without discrimination to every adult and child, whatever their gender, sexual preference, race, religion, politics, achievements, crimes, miseries, etc.

I believe the innocent baby who became a candy thief, the gentle mother who spanked her toddler for disobedience, and the devoted father who incarcerated his son for grabbing another child's toys, will always be the same people they've always been. Their thoughts, attitudes, and behaviors may shift in response to their internal and external circumstances but, at the core, they are making choices on their own behalf. This leads me to my central question about the time we often refer to as the 'terrible-twos' – why are the children and their parents behaving so 'badly'?

If you ask the parents, they'll probably tell you the child is the problem. In my profession, appointment books and wait lists are crammed with Moms and Dads seeking help to understand and manage their misbehaving offspring. The more 'enlightened' ones may consider this to be a transitory phase of childhood, and want advice on short-term damage control – "What should we do when she shrieks her head off after we tell her it's bedtime?" Others are more psychoanalytically perturbed - "Yesterday, he took a knife from the kitchen table and pretended to stab himself in the chest. Is this some kind of death wish?" Many are simply hard-working parents who pick up their child from day-care and have little in reserve to deal with shenanigans of a Tasmanian Devil. One way or another, they are all perplexed and frustrated.

It's the time when the Self needs to know it has the resources and the ability to take charge of its own destiny, to experience the power that lies on the inside.

The Omnipotent Narcissist

And so are the children. The only difference is that their behavior is not only understandable, it's also perfectly natural. For them this is a pivotal period in the quest for separation and individuation. It's the time when the Self needs to know it has the resources and the ability to take charge of its own destiny, to experience the power that lies on the inside. Unrestrained by moral evaluations and social conventions, the child is ready to strike out for Liberty - but to Hell with Equality, Fraternity and all that other stuff. This isn't the calculating agenda of a psychopath; it's the self-indulgence of a committed narcissist. The message to the world is "Here I am, look at me, I'm the greatest. I'll take what I want when I want it, so stay out of the way." Adults who were never allowed to experience such narcissism in their own childhood are often repulsed by this presentation and feel the urge to 'teach that kid some humility.'

But this is a transitory phase that is critical in two ways. On the one hand, it's a planned opportunity for the child to experience the raw indomitable Spirit that lies at the core of the Self. On the other it is an opportunity for the world to acknowledge that Self, and speak back with a firm, gentle and caring voice. To use a common metaphor, it's a 'testing of the waters.' If the water seems gentle and enticing, the swimmer may set out with unquestioning and naive assurance. If it's cold, rejecting and treacherous, the would-be adventurer may decide to recoil from the prospect and settle for the safety of life on the shore. If the water is warm and welcoming, and there's an experienced and enthusiastic lifeguard available to encourage the beginner, while teaching the necessary skills and pointing out the potential hazards, the novice will confidently set out in a relatively safe and self-responsible way. This, I believe, is the key to understanding and dealing with the "terrible twos."

For parents and caregivers, this can be a monumental challenge. According to the universal parenting handbook, they are obliged to 'socialize' their children, making it clear which behaviors are acceptable and which are not. In western cultures, most parents believe it's also their job to teach the difference between right and wrong in accordance with the prevailing morality. Understandably they want to be proud of their offspring and not be shown up in public.

How can all this be accomplished without confronting and suppressing an unrestrained Self that seems intent on sabotaging the entire project? How can this time be transformed from a tedious, and potentially injurious, power struggle into an exciting learning opportunity?

Well, it isn't easy. In the first place the adults must be aware of what's happening within the child's experience and recognize this as a critical time in the development of the Self. This does not mean they should simply back off and let Hell run rampant. All children need to know what the world expects and acquire the skills necessary in adapting to a particular family, society and culture. Above all they need to learn how to bring their inherent need for connection into their relationships with other human beings. The art of 'good enough' parenting is to work with both sides of the equation; to teach the acceptable behaviors while remaining responsive to a naive Self that is attempting to explore and express its own inner resources. The secret lies in the ability of the parent to bring both aspects together in responding to the child's behavior. Saying 'no' and imposing appropriate consequences does not necessitate the withdrawal of love and caring. Even the parent who is momentarily angry can reconnect when the upset has subsided; this is all part of the learning continuum. As a general rule, the 'good enough' parent will act in the best interests of the child, but there will be times when frustration triggers emotions that interrupt the flow of this intention. This is not a problem unless the intensity and duration of the slippage fractures the relationship and inflicts emotional or physical injury upon the child. This is particularly serious where the parent who has failed to deal with his or her own developmental injuries loses control. In such circumstances, it is the responsibility of that parent to seek help and, if necessary, the child should be removed from the danger zone.

Where the interruptions are transitory and tolerable for the child, the critical factor is to bring the Self back into the equation by attending to and acknowledging, the child's feelings. Inviting the child to share his or her experience and accurately mirroring the responses can achieve this. The misbehaving youngster who is carried to his room screaming, "I hate you, I hate you, you're bad, I hate you," is not immediately interested in learning how to express his or her emotions more appropriately. This may not be the kind of stuff most parents want to hear, but the feelings are real nonetheless. An angry parent may react with punishment, intent on teaching the kid what a bad parent is really like – the old "I'll show you" stance. The door slams and the struggle escalates until the superior power of the adult finally wins the day. Later, after both combatants have cooled off, the incident sinks into the past and life returns to normal. But all is not forgotten, nor forgiven. The parent may have confirmed his or her place of authority but the sense of being hated lingers on. The child who has submitted to that authority may think twice before committing the same crime again, but the feelings of powerlessness and resentment remain. While the memory may fade, left in this way the incident will become locked into the parent-child relationship – unacknowledged and unresolved.

The real tragedy is that a wonderful learning opportunity has been lost in battle. The parent who takes the time to reflect on his or her feelings will recognize them for what they really were – a reaction to not being loved, appreciated and respected. No need to bring in an Attachment Therapist; the locus of the problem is then owned by the adult. The parent is now free to be curious about the experiences of a three-year old who wants to feel powerful and omnipotent in a world that seems intent on repressing his or her enthusiasm. The child's hatred and rage may have been directed at the parent, but they stem from the unbearable frustration of being controlled. With this understanding, parent and child can reconnect and the learning can begin.

In a quiet moment and settled space, the 'good enough' parent can be fully present with the child with no agenda other than to be curious, listen and reflect:

"When I was upset and took you to your room this morning, you seemed very angry with me too."

"I hate you when you do that. I hate you when you're bad."

"Yes, you were screaming and yelling. You must have been very angry."

"I only wanted to play with Molly ... I wasn't going to hurt her."

"So, you didn't like it when I told you to leave her alone."

"I only wanted to play and you wouldn't let me."

"So, when I grabbed your arm, you felt angry with me."

"You hurt me."

"I hurt your arm."

"You hurt me all over."

"Yes, I can see you're crying now."

"I don't like it when you're mad at me."

"I don't like it either. Where does it hurt?"

"Right here in my tummy."

The thing to notice about this dialogue is that no attempt is being made to resolve a problem. Nor is the parent trying to explain, justify or apologize for any actions taken. No changes are called for, and no promises are made on either side. This is not a teaching exercise; it's an opportunity for the child to explore and express his or her feelings. This provides an outlet for the 'rage' that might otherwise continue to simmer on the inside, but more profoundly, it acknowledges the Self as an integral part of the parent-child relationship. This will only happen if the reconciled Self of the adult is free to become fully present and engaged.

I don't know about you, but as a child, I was never asked about my feelings. Even though I felt generally loved and cared for, I was left wondering how people could possibly love me if they didn't even know me. As time went on I learned to keep my inner world a secret for fear that anyone who found out who I really was, would withdraw his or her affection. Up to the age of ten, I was known for my horrendous temper tantrums. Rather than deal with the fury, family members would back off and, for a brief time, I would get my own way. Next would come the isolation and I would sink into guilt and remorse. Eventually I would come creeping back, doing whatever was necessary to gain reassurance and reconnection. Those who wanted to teach me a lesson would deliberately try to make this difficult, but with each of them, I learned the most effective ways to manipulate my way back in. In this way I was able to stay 'attached' while keeping my Self at a distance – a skill I continue to use whenever the circumstances seem appropriate.

Given the opportunity, all kids moving through this developmental phase will try to control their parents one way or another. They want to move under their own steam, but they also want to know the adults are there to provide attention, service and security on demand. This applies as much as the child who learns how to please the parents as it does to the youngster who fights every inch of the way. If the parents allow themselves to be controlled in this manner, the child's transitory narcissism will turn into an enduring sense of entitlement. Other people will continue to be regarded as servants in the mansion of self-indulgence rather than as distinct and separate beings with their own feelings, hopes and wishes. Children will not develop this 'other-awareness' unless the servants speak back by establishing their own autonomy and revealing their own unique needs and qualities as individuals.

This awareness makes it possible for children to take the next step toward creating personal relationships based upon mutual recognition and respect. By not automatically getting their own way, they come to recognize their parents as separate and purposeful individuals in their own right. This is more about defining and sustaining personal boundaries than simply enforcing arbitrary rules. Of course children should be required to behave in accordance with set standards of acceptability, but learning to acknowledge and respect parental boundaries is far more important for the development of a separate and individuated sense of Self.

Parents who like to share their innermost thoughts and feelings with their two-year old infants might just as well be talking to the family pit-bull.

The first rudimentary task is for parents to establish and maintain their boundaries in a consistent, caring and non-negotiable manner. Over time, as children become progressively able to sense the feelings of others, they can tolerate greater degrees of boundary flexibility. By coming to understand that "yes" this morning may be "no" this afternoon, they learn that our internal experiences are constantly shifting, and close relationships involve ongoing sensitivity between Self and Other. This important developmental shift – referred to as 'perspective taking' or 'role-taking' – is facilitated through the willingness of the parents to share their own inner experiences while remaining curious about the subject experiences of the child. Since accurate perspective taking involves complex cognitive processes, parents who like to share their innermost thoughts and feelings with their two-year old infants might just as well be talking to the family pit-bull. The intentions might be admirable but unless the child is able to hear and understand, the exercise is pointless – at least for the child.

And this raises a very important issue. Much as I have cautioned against viewing children through the lens of one theory or another, it is important for all parents to have some basic understanding of the developmental process. Insisting that the same two-year old share his favorite toy with his baby sister can be like asking that same pit-bull to offer its ham shank to a visiting poodle. Taking away the bone and chaining up Rambo for his selfishness will not teach him to be more hospitable in the future. You can be sure that handing over the coveted bone to Twickypoo will do nothing to enhance the quality of the canine relationship. Of course, you could always talk to Rambo afterwards, and appeal to his conscience by explaining the importance of sharing and fair play – that should do the trick.

I don't really mean to imply that two-year olds are 'animalistic,' totally insensitive to the needs and feelings of others. I have already described how even newborns can respond empathetically to the distress of another infant. We are talking about a specific period of development in which children are challenged to explore and experience the deepest resources of the Self. Children who are supported in this task and are taught how to channel those resources in a socially viable way will move forward in the world with confidence. No matter what life has in store, these children will always know they have what it takes to act on their own behalf. When adversity strikes, they can always return to home base, lick their wounds, and come back for more. This is the foundation of personal autonomy and 'resilience'- not the protection that comes from building effective defenses, but the inner strength that can only be drawn from Self-reliance.

For the time being, this task is enough. At this point, children are not ready to consider the complexity of values and beliefs that make up the adult's determination of right and wrong. In the world of the child what feels good is right and what feels bad is wrong. It's that simple. I have been known to argue that this yardstick is more authentic than the contrived and conflicted moralities that plague this planet, but I'll leave that for another time. What needs to be understood is that children who are inebriated by narcissism are not ready to engage in moral reasoning; this comes later. Over the years, I've heard so much nonsense from parents and professionals who seem determined to teach their particular version of kindness, justice and fair play to kids who are obsessed with their own self-indulgence. When the youngsters fail to respond, their teachers are often inclined to punish the transgressions. This may result in more morally acceptable behavior, but the methods employed deliver a savage blow to the child's burgeoning sense of Self.

In the world of the child what feels good is right and what feels bad is wrong. It's that simple.

If you're familiar with the ideas put forward by such influential theorists as Jean Piaget and Lawrence Kohlberg, you might assume that I'm reiterating their stance that moral development is a linear procession, with each stage constructed on the back of its predecessor. This is not the case. I believe all children are inherently relational and sensitive to the feelings and needs of others. During this 'narcissistic' phase of development these qualities may be temporarily overwhelmed, but they are always there and ready to play their part. Even at the peak of their most demanding and obnoxious episodes, young children will usually back down when they sense another person is in distress. If this does not occur and the child persistently ignores or fuels that distress, there is good reason to believe that some significant bonding injury has interrupted the developmental process. This idea that, in the natural course of events, all aspects of the Self remain open to learning and expression is closer to Stern's view than the perspective generally taken by the classical 'stage' theorists. The point for parents, caretakers and teachers to remember is that they are always dealing with the whole child, regardless of the specific circumstances and where that youngster happens to be on the developmental continuum.

Full Esteem Ahead

For over fifty years the notion of self-esteem has maintained a ubiquitous presence in child development, education, and parenting literature. There was a time when obedience and successful school performance were thought to be the reasons why children would feel good about themselves. Now the common assumption seems to be that kids with high self-esteem are more likely to be obedient and academically successful. On the other side, low self-esteem has been identified as a significant contributor to many youth-related problems, including substance abuse, bullying, juvenile crime, eating disorders, depression and teenage suicide. Using research terminology, this shift from dependent to independent variable has given rise to a plethora of prescriptions designed specifically to enhance the value a child attributes to himself or herself.

The point for parents, caretakers and teachers to remember is that they are always dealing with the whole child, regardless of the specific circumstances and where that youngster happens to be on the developmental continuum.

The trouble is, most of these strategies pay absolutely no attention to the 'Self' the child is supposed to feel good about. From birth onwards, the general idea seems to be that if we focus on the positives, pouring on praise, points and prizes for preferred performances, the child will internalize these evaluations and go on to make us proud. However, unless these external appraisals are authentic expressions, congruent with the child's internal reality, the real Selves of all participants are excluded from the action. The negotiated images traded between adult and child merge into a masquerade of impression management – loving parent and ideal child. These are the conditions that create and reinforce the 'false self,' a projected image constructed from the desires and expectations of others. Much has been written about how the child comes to disregard, or even despise the Self on the inside, but I believe the Self of the adult is also sacrificed in the quest to create what 'should be,' rather than what 'is.' In other words, despite all the smiles, back-patting and good feelings, there is no direct contact between one Self and an Other. The result is simple manipulation.

The 'bad-boy'- 'good-boy' approach addresses the wishes of the parents and offers no attention to the subjective experience of the child.

In dealing with the narcissistic acting-out of a two-year-old, parents may be tempted to compensate for their negative feelings and responses by 'over-mirroring' the more acceptable behaviors. While this might be understandable, the 'bad-boy'- 'good-boy' approach addresses the wishes of the parents and offers no attention to the subjective experience of the child. Of course children need to know when their parents are pleased and displeased, but unless the Self of the child is brought into the process, the chances are that this externally imposed dichotomy will become entrenched in the youngster's psyche. From an object-relations perspective, the persistent

As the external voice of the parent becomes the inner voice of the child, the youngster will continue to be dependent upon the approval of others in order to maintain a valued sense of self.

use of this strategy can effectively arrest the developmental process by preventing the child from moving toward object constancy. Even more profoundly, the child's struggle to match the parental ideals may result in the denial and depreciation of the 'real' Self on the inside. As the external voice of the parent becomes the inner voice of the child, the youngster will continue to be dependent upon the approval of others in order to maintain a valued sense of self. Eventually, the authentic Self will become buried beneath increasing overlays of judgments and pretensions, unseen, unheard and, to all intents and purposes, unacceptable.

The basic foundations of self-esteem are not difficult to understand; in fact most have already been identified in previous discussions. At the very core children need to know they exist as separate beings and that their inner experiences are real and legitimate. Taking the time to be curious, and mirror without judgment, is not only an acknowledgment of that separateness but is also an affirmation of the child's inherent 'rightness'. The esteem of young children is not built

The esteem of young children is not built upon positive thoughts but upon good feelings – an inner sense of well being that comes from being recognized and cared for by loving adults.

upon positive thoughts but upon good feelings – an inner sense of well being that comes from being recognized and cared for by loving adults. These foundations are energetic and experienced in the body. When words and thoughts come into the picture, it is important that they be congruent with these pre-existing feelings. In this way the child is able to construct an internalized self-image that blends all facets of experience into an integrated and meaningful whole.

Throughout this process, the most essential element is that the internal feelings of rightness and well being remain as the central points of reference. This does not imply that children should never feel badly about themselves. On the contrary, such feelings play a vital role in the development of self-management, integrity and self-responsibility. Becoming true to one's Self is very different from learning how to conform to external judgments and prescriptions. The words and behaviors may appear to be similar but people who are motivated by their own sense of being possess a quality of integrity and purpose that cannot be adjusted by changing the rules, or reclaimed through atonement and apology. With this in mind, I do not believe parents and educators are obliged to teach children the difference between 'right' and 'wrong' - this is already known. What children need is to learn how to access and express their inherent humanity in a world of competing truths and warring factions.

In their book, *The Manual for Life*, Bennet Wong and Jock McKeen make an astute distinction between feelings of shame and the experience of guilt. According to their definitions shame is a natural internal state that recognizes the personal fallibility in all of us; recognition of not being all we could be. Guilt on the other hand is a "complex of feelings involving regret, self-recrimination, depression, anxiety, and fear of punishment, arising from having transgressed some code of behavior originally defined externally". (p144). In their view guilt is highly valued in western societies as a means of maintaining social control whereas many Asian cultures consider shame, like mindfulness and empathy, to be a wholesome state of consciousness. In terms of the current discussion, the most significant feature of this distinction is that shame relates directly to the Self whereas guilt relates to external judgments and consequences.

In this sense shame paves the way toward self-responsibility while guilt is more about accountability to external authority. Although we often use the word shame as a verb – to shame a child, or an external pronouncement – "You should be ashamed of yourself," these are contrary to the meanings suggested by Wong and McKeen. Shame is a personal experience that relates to the integrity of the emerging Self and the resources for reaffirming that integrity lie within. By contrast guilt is the impersonal experience of being judged and is ameliorated through external forgiveness.

> *Shame paves the way toward self-responsibility while guilt is more about accountability to external authority. Shame is a personal experience that relates to the integrity of the emerging Self and the resources for reaffirming that integrity lie within. By contrast guilt is the impersonal experience of being judged and is ameliorated through external forgiveness.*

Over the years I have worked with many children crippled by guilt and self-recrimination, but only rarely have I encountered a child whose primary concern is with his or her sense of personal integrity. Such children are more likely to be sad and reflective than depressed and fearful. In therapy the task is to support them in exploring their own strength in becoming all they could be. There is nothing to fix or remediate and since they already see themselves at the centre of their own lives, we are not concerned with teaching self-responsibility. What they need are affirmations of what they already know, not contrived evaluations of what they do. Their sadness is real as they are real, and working with them can be a truly human experience for both parties. And yes, these kids also need to know the rules and learn how to live within the framework of the social order.

Perhaps the time has come for us to reconsider our cultural obsession with high self-esteem. Maybe it's okay for a child to feel just ordinary, accepting that others might be brighter or more talented. Is it possible for us to incorporate the virtue of true humility into a competitive society that appears to recognize only success and achievement? What prevents us from encouraging our children to take pleasure in the accomplishment of everyday tasks rather than spur them on to ever increasing standards of achievement – and self-esteem test scores? If they fail to meet our expectations surely that's more about us than about them. In addition, if they feel badly about themselves, so be it. We can always be there to listen to their story, acknowledge their feelings and support them in exploring the options. At very least we can adopt the mandate Hippocrates supposedly established for physicians – first do no harm. As in medicine, the harm we do is seldom obvious.

The Autonomous Self is its Own Reward

To a large extent feeling good about ourselves is based upon a belief that we are in charge of our lives. If this belief is established in early childhood we grow up making our own choices and taking responsibility for our actions. Alternatively, if we grow up believing that others control our behavior, we develop little faith in our innate abilities and attribute our successes and failures to chance and circumstance. In psychology this is often referred to as "internal locus of control" – a term coined by social learning theorist J.B. Rotter in the 1950's and exemplified through the work of researchers such as Edward Deci at the University of Rochester. To illustrate how this works I will refer to a modest study conducted with three colleagues during my graduate school days.

Given access to the students at two local high schools, we selected a group of subjects who liked to solve puzzles. The puzzle we offered was called 'wordplay' and involved sorting out a multitude of scrambled letters into specific words, sentences and paragraphs.

All our subjects had demonstrated high interest by working on these puzzles in their own time, without any encouragement for at least an hour. We then randomly assigned our solvers to one of four groups. In the first group, subjects were paid two dollars for each puzzle solved. In the second, they were supervised by an 'active' observer who recorded each success and congratulated the solver. In the third group, a 'passive' observer who offered no response for performance provided the supervision. In the final fourth, the 'control' group, they were simply left alone to play. All groups were given one hour with the instruction they could continue on if they so wished.

We were not particularly surprised by the initial outcomes. Students who were paid for their efforts were by far the most successful with a completion rate well beyond the baseline established during pre-testing. They also remained the longest – some were obviously prepared to stay all night if given the opportunity. Those who were provided with active supervision also scored significantly higher than the pre-tested levels and most continued beyond the one-hour period. Those who were passively supervised also performed above the baseline but there was great variability among members of this group. Some scored very highly while others seemed to flag and left as soon as the obligatory hour was up. The control group performed as expected. Their scores were consistent with the pre-test level and their average time was just under two hours.

Four days later, we brought all our subjects back and repeated the original procedure by inviting them to work with puzzles for as long as they wished with no variation in conditions – no monetary rewards, no feedback and no supervision. The results clearly confirmed the findings of other researchers in the field. The performance and longevity of subjects who had previously received financial rewards fell dramatically. Compared with their pre-test scores, they demonstrated a significant loss of interest in puzzle solving. A similar effect was found in the actively supervised group, although a small number actually scored higher and stayed longer. In the passively supervised group the scores were marginally lower than the pre-test results, but only two of these subjects stayed for more than an hour. Subjects in the 'control' group who, again, stayed with the activity for almost two hours recorded the only stable scores.

Some General Conclusions and Implications

Out of respect for my supervisors and colleagues, I need to acknowledge that this is a very brief and inadequate synopsis of what was to become a very thorough and complex research project that produced two Ph.D. dissertations – neither of them belonging to me. As with all pilot studies the more detailed and intriguing questions emerged from an analysis of the preliminary data and subsequent investigations. My primary concern here is with our overall conclusion: Giving people external reasons to do what they already want to do can effectively undermine their internal or intrinsic motivation. If you take the time to read Edward Deci's book *Intrinsic Motivation*, published in 1975 you will see how this overall effect is subject to many 'ifs, ands and buts,' yet the basic principle remains to be considered by all who seek to motivate or modify the behavior of others – children included. One explanation for the findings in our own

If it is within their nature to seek connection, live 'moral' lives and emulate their parents, why do we feel the need to secure their love, teach them right from wrong and prescribe the pathway for their lives?

study is that the subjects who demonstrated the greatest loss of intrinsic motivation were those who became focused on the external 'reasons' for their behavior. In this regard it's interesting to note that money had by far the most significant negative effect – a sign of our culture, perhaps.

So why am I taking the time to drag out research from the 1970's to illustrate my point? Well the reason is that those who now promote and sponsor psychological research have not shown any particular interest in examining our innate capacities for self-determination. I wonder why? My point is that, despite all the talk about humanistic and holistic psychology, our basic educational and parenting practices continue to focus primarily upon the use of external contingencies to ensure the 'successful' development of our children. Yet if we stop to consider even the broadest implications of this research, we would have to examine the possibility that these child-rearing methods are crude and potentially harmful.

If we begin with the assumption that children come into this world intrinsically motivated to become all they can be, surely our primary task is to guide and support this process, rather than to make it happen. If it is within their nature to seek connection, live 'moral' lives and emulate their parents, why do we feel the need to secure their love, teach them right from wrong and prescribe the pathway for their lives? What a strange twist of irony that the harder we try the more they may conform, but the less they will want to. Can it be that, in our desire to see them succeed, we risk turning their hopes into obligations and their dreams into nightmares? To consider this possibility doesn't mean we should immediately stop offering our children encouragement, teaching them the ropes and lowering the boom when their behavior is unacceptable. One of the clear conclusions to be drawn from the research is that it isn't the external stimulus per se that impacts motivation, but the individual's perception of that event. This brings us back to where our attention should really be focused – the subjective experience of the child.

For example if a five-dollar reward is given for mowing the lawn, the child may perceive this as recognition for a job well done, a chance to go to the movies, or an attempt to control his or her behavior. In the first case, the reward will serve to enhance feelings of competence, confidence and self-determination. In the second, there is no real connection between the behavior and the reward. And in the third, it will be perceived as an external 'reason' for having to do something. While the observable outcomes may appear similar – increased willingness to mow the lawn – the motivational implications are very different. To stretch a point, we might expect that, in the first condition the child will actually find pleasure in the work, while in the second and third, he or she will end up like most of us - working for others, demanding to be paid for our efforts and throwing in the towel if we feel ripped off. And what about the child who is promised that trip to Disneyland for an extended period of 'good' behavior or the achievement of some distant goal? Well, unless this catchall reward is the culmination of feedback given for specific behaviors, the chances are that the big pay-off will draw both parent and child into endless negotiations with the prospects of success or failure constantly dangling in the background. The good behaviors and school achievements are no longer valued for their own sake but only for their potential to claim the anticipated compensation.

Working with this general proposition, it's not difficult to imagine what the effects of negative feedback, sanctions and punishment will have on intrinsic motivation. Children may attempt to match parental expectations in order to avoid such outcomes, but feeling controlled and resentful they will almost certainly end up devaluing the behavior and seek alternative possibilities for self-determination. As we all know this can lead to resistance and eventually, outright rebellion. We should not be surprised to learn that the research clearly confirms that these external conditions are by far the most effective in suppressing intrinsic motivation.

In any given situation, how a particular child responds to an external stimulus or event will be largely determined by his or her learning history up to that point. Children who have been encouraged to be internally focused through their early development will naturally assume this stance in dealing with the responses of others toward them. They will accept rewards as competence feedback in pursuing their own interests and purposes. Possessing a reasonably solid sense of Self, they will not be devastated by negative messages, or thrown off course by external manipulation. Conversely, children who have no faith in their own interiority have only the outside world to identify and confirm their rightness and their place in the scheme of things. Their feelings are governed by the responses of others - good, bad or indifferent - and in their view, whatever happens is beyond their control. In many cases such children have been exposed to inadequate or negative feedback and come to believe that their actions have little or no impact on external events. In the extreme case this is often referred to as a state of 'learned helplessness'; a place where the last vestiges of intrinsic motivation have been effectively eradicated.

It is important to recognize that most children are both intrinsically and extrinsically motivated. The interesting question is whether a child's position on this continuum can be influenced by current experiences and, according to the research findings, the answer is clearly in the affirmative. Children who believe in their own capacities for self-determination can be persuaded to give up this stance when exposed to conditions that emphasize the importance of external rewards and sanctions. Alternatively those who have little belief in their own powers of self-determination can be convinced otherwise through a sensitively designed approach that links their behavior to particular outcomes or consequences. This connection can only be made through constant references to the child's sense of Self and affirmations of his or her self-efficacy. A caring adult who recognizes these potentials can be guided by only one central point of reference – the subjective experience of the child. Only by understanding the child's perspective is it possible to predict whether any reward or disciplinary measure will enhance or depreciate the youngster's sense of self-determination and self-responsibility. For parents the issue is very simple – get to know your kids.

> *Only by understanding the child's perspective is it possible to predict whether any reward or disciplinary measure will enhance or depreciate the youngster's sense of self-determination and self-responsibility.*

Real Play is Self-Motivated

Perhaps the most difficult obstacle to understanding the world of a child is that of convincing the rational mind to embrace the fictions and fantasies of developmental play. When watching children at play, adults are inclined to assume a distinctly egocentric perspective by noticing how so much time seems to be spent taking on adult roles and mannerisms while acting out imaginary adult scenarios. This view of children's play as a process of socialization, a rehearsal for adulthood, is not only shallow and narrow, but offers yet another example of how we have chosen to ignore the subjective experiences of childhood – including our own. It has also given rise to the belief that we can facilitate the developmental process by providing children with stuffed animals, plastic warriors, Ronald McDonald playgrounds and those grotesque "Theme Parks' that leave little or nothing to the creative imagination. Sadly, this is because so many of us were 'taught' how to play by well meaning adults.

In effect what happens is very similar to the process described in the above discussion on intrinsic motivation. In both cases the child's attention is drawn away from his or her natural inclinations on the inside to become focused on the external stimuli. In the child's mind the reasons for playing, along with the associated feelings, become attributed to outside sources. For example the statement "I'm always happy when I get to play with my crayons" may be replaced by "Mickey Mouse makes me happy." This shift may go unnoticed because when our children are happy, we are happy too. But this is not play, by any stretch of the imagination.

In its natural form imaginative play is an integral ingredient in the development of a purposeful Self. Unfettered by external demands and expectations, the naive infant comes into this world saying "Here I am. I'm here to play" and subsequently asks, "Who wants to play with me?" In its earliest and most primitive form, play is concerned with the manipulation of objects, real and imagined. In the child's first encounters with the physical world, this is an exploratory adventure involving all the senses. The properties of objects are examined by seeing, hearing, touching and through direct manipulation. Sometimes referred to as 'sensory motor play,' this provides not only cognitive stimulation but also the pleasure that comes from being able to influence external events. In this way the core Self confirms its place in the object world and begins to discover its own sense of efficacy. These are elements common to all forms of play throughout life.

According to the conventional wisdom of developmental psychology, this exploratory play is 'facilitated' through stimulation provided by parents. Personally I find this assertion misleading, and to the degree it implies that the parent must be the initiator, potentially harmful. If we believe the infant simply responds to the actions of the parent, we have taken the first critical step in shifting from an internal to an external frame of reference. With the infant in the passenger seat, the onus is upon adults to determine whether they are under-stimulating or over-stimulating, based upon their interpretations of the infant's responses. The problem is not so much in their behavior as in the attitude that lies behind their actions – an attitude that is communicated to the child energetically. Even if the parent sensitively adjusts stimulation levels according to the child's responses, the assumption that the adult leads the way imposes itself on an emerging Self that is seeking to explore the parameters of its influence in the world.

Not only is this an anathema to my beliefs about the essential needs of the Self, it is also contrary to my experience of playing with infants. Even during the first few months of life babies are very capable of communicating their needs and initiating playful interactions. The old standard game of peek-a-boo, for example, can be a response to a baby's intermittent gaze and the pleasure expressed by the infant can be mirrored to create a sense of mutual fun. I'm not suggesting the adult should never initiate playful activity. Relationships are based upon mutuality and, by definition, interactive play is a back-and-forth affair. Nor am I discounting the role of the parent in offering new opportunities for excitement or adjusting stimulation to optimal levels. Together these elements are all part of what Daniel Stern refers to as a 'mutually regulating dyadic system'. My concern here is with the significance of play as a child-directed activity and a foundation for the development of personal autonomy.

Whatever the infant learns from the earliest play experiences is carried into the time when the cognitive or 'existential' aspects of the Self come into play (pun intended). This is particularly evident during the 'narcissistic' period when the child is seeking to experience the sense of omnipotence that will become the core resource on the inside. At this time play becomes an opportunity to explore aspects of the Self where the usual conditions and restraints don't apply and 'reality' is infinitely negotiable. Through play the child can experience being the author of his or her own stories, making it possible for body and mind to explore new realms of imagination and creativity. This is also a time when parents are most likely to become concerned about the apparent disregard for the consensual reality of the adult world and step in to redirect the child toward a more acceptable or understandable world-view. Certainly there will be times when a child's play gets out of hand and intervention is called for, but the creative, imaginative and emotional expressions, however unreal or bizarre they might appear, should be recognized for what they really are – explorations of the parameters of the Self.

Eventually the time will come when the child will seek to test out his or her Self-creations against the 'real world,' usually around the age of three, and one way or another that world will speak back, not only through the parents

Through play the child can experience being the author of his or her own stories, making it possible for body and mind to explore new realms of imagination and creativity.

but through whoever the child encounters. This process, known as 'rapprochement,' involves bringing internal fantasies into harmony with external reality. Although psychologists have traditionally considered this to be a definitive developmental stage, the 'open' model proposed by Daniel Stern makes much more sense to me. My own experience fully supports the notion that rapprochement occurs throughout life whenever we take our existing self-view into new or strange circumstances.

I well remember the difficulties I encountered when I took my raw and rigid working-class identity and attitudes into the placid pastures of a middle class English University. I was determined not to become one of 'them,' and made my differences known at every opportunity. Apart from the odd skirmish over a few pints of ale, nobody seemed particularly interested and I was left to drift around with a disgruntled group of self-indulgent deviants. Since my own childhood narcissism was never really supported, I had no solid sense of Self to fall back on, and I learned how to cover up my lingering feelings of insecurity through postured acts of assertiveness, rebellion and the occasional temper tantrum. Now this stuff was getting in the way. I began to see how I was sabotaging my own aspirations, and in an unprecedented act of reverse rebellion, I took my clarinet and joined the University Jazz Club. Sharing this passion with the enemy, I began to carve out a niche for myself on the other side. Later when I returned to my home community, some of my old buddies were convinced I'd sacrificed my soul to the oppressors, but I really hadn't. In fact I was beginning to discover a world in which my spirit had never been freer: I had created a playground for myself in the parking lot of academia. Finally I came to understand the old saying, 'real freedom is wearing your galoshes even if your mother tells you to.'

When children are allowed to move through their primitive narcissism with sensitivity and tolerance, their play moves naturally toward the inclusion of others. Activities become increasingly co-creative as uncharted realities are negotiated and explored. Free from external prescriptions, children are able to experiment with an infinite array of identities and possibilities. Roles can be taken on and discarded without responsibilities or sanctions, and every action can reflect the exuberance of the unbound Self. Unless the 'other' reality imposes to reject or castigate this imaginative design, the process is one in which the Self of each child becomes progressively enhanced, elaborated and differentiated.

Such play is not simply infantile fantasy; it's a process of developmental integration. Body movements are brought together with feeling and thinking states. As an integral aspect of rapprochement, fantasy and the external world are gradually brought into harmonious, or at least manageable, connection. This is a time when children begin to understand that others also have inner lives, similar to, and different from their own. Social-perspective-taking and role-taking ability are the outcomes of the imagination as it becomes progressively focused and grounded in the shared reality of relationships. Simple connections and dependencies are transformed into more complex configurations of empathy and mutuality, expressed through acts of caring and sharing. Through play the world of objects becomes increasingly personalized as the child's attention shifts from narcissistic self-involvement to a curiosity about how others are thinking and feeling. If adults are able to resist the temptation to

Through play the world of objects becomes increasingly personalized as the child's attention shifts from narcissistic self-involvement to a curiosity about how others are thinking and feeling.

impose themselves, the child's inherent human qualities will naturally extrapolate into the 'moral' values and social attitudes that form the foundation of any caring community. Values and beliefs specific to a given society or culture can then be offered to a curious and receptive listener.

Play is Not For Amusement

Allowing a child to play can be a significant challenge to parents who confuse childhood play with the adult concept of 'amusement.' The problem is that children who are passively or even actively, drawn into amusing activities can become hooked on the external stimulation. Television and video games are classic examples of how easily this addiction can be acquired. I'm not suggesting children should be denied access to these staples of our culture, but they should never be considered as play or even substitutes for play. All children need some form of external stimulation, but activities that directly engage the child's creative and imaginative potentials are less likely to create dependency and serve to enhance the natural course of self-directed development. In this regard books are always preferable to movies, finger-painting beats out coloring books, and modeling clay is infinitely superior to dump trucks and Barbie dolls.

But play, '*real*' play, must always be initiated and controlled by children themselves. Even those rare adults who are able to enter a child's world of fantasy can never become fully qualified playmates, however much they might try. And that's the way it should be. When adults take up their rightful position on the outside, the young cavalier is free to embark upon the incredible adventures and believe in the unbelievable, always knowing that he or she can return to a pair of safe hands, warm milk and chocolate-chip cookies. The most adults can do is to watch from a distance with acceptance and appreciation. Their essential role is to grant opportunities for children to play without the imposition of structure and with little or no facilitation. Their priceless reward is the privilege of observing an unbridled Spirit defying the boundaries of possibility, before the 'real' world imposes its shackles of rationality and conformity. They should never watch with the belief that it should be all about laughter and happy times in Turnip Land. By its very nature, play generates conditions in which every image, thought and emotion can be stretched to the limit. Joy, frustration, anger, despair, sadness, and fear are all amplified well beyond acceptable adult levels but this is what the learning is all about. There may be many times when the observing adult is tempted to intervene, but unless there are obvious reasons to the contrary, it should be the child's decision to step out of the arena when the going is too much to handle.

What Happened at School Today?

One choice a child is not empowered to make is whether or not to go to school. When I began writing this book, I realized that, sooner or later, I would have to address the topic of education, and I balked at the prospect. My major dilemma was, and still is, that I honestly don't know where to start. While I found it relatively easy to consider the impact of the health care system on early child development, a state governed educational system is a far more insidious monster. What could I possibly say about a legally imposed regime that holds children captive for over ten years before pushing them into serving the economic, political and institutional interests of the state? I'm not talking about some distant totalitarian power – I'm referring to the state operated educational systems in North America, Europe and throughout the developed world. I suppose I could always dig up isolated programs that appear to support the natural development of the child, but these are rare exceptions that for the most part operate outside the mainstream network. Having spent so many years working in and around the fortresses of institutional learning, I'm afraid my perceptions and attitudes have become irrevocably tarnished. I am now firmly of the opinion that nothing will change until primary caregivers, individually and collectively, reclaim responsibility for what happens to their children in the name of 'education.' And once again, the individual pathway appears the most viable.

From the grade schools to the universities, educational programs have been converted into standardized job training packages, instilling the value of competition from the outset and channeling kids into prescribed career pathways at the earliest possible opportunity.

In my view, schools and their bureaucracies have done to human consciousness what churches and their religious orders have done to human spirituality. Both have taken the most noble of human quests – to be curious, to seek meaning, to find expression, to be connected, to love, to touch the divine – and twisted them into grotesque configurations of power, control and obedience. Both draw their power from a base of fear and punishment - from the fear of failure and rejection to the prospect of eternal damnation. Both are founded upon an underlying attitude of mistrust; a belief that once beyond the vigilant eyes of authority, the masses will naturally sink into sin, deviance and anarchy. Both are pyramids of authoritarianism through which information and privilege are selectively handed down from each level to the one below. And both are carefully engineered to service the interests of those who wield the power from the top – whether in the name of reason or the name of God.

If you have been lulled into thinking of compulsory education as an essential public service, take a look at how the declining power of governments has shifted the focus of education from preserving the social order to servicing the profit margins of the corporate world. From the grade schools to the universities, educational programs have been converted into standardized job training packages, instilling the value of competition from the outset and channeling kids into prescribed career pathways at the earliest possible opportunity. You may also notice how educational establishments at all levels, have become increasingly dependent upon corporate sponsorship, and the proverbial piper is calling a hideous tune. What we call 'education' is not about curiosity and the joy of learning, but about compliance with the agenda of the investors. It's not that this has suddenly come along to contaminate some pure version of educational philosophy and practice. Whatever the Greeks did or didn't do, our educational establishments, both public and private, have always been set up to satisfy the prevailing social, religious, political and economic elite. The problem is that such systems have become increasingly anachronistic, particularly in societies where the causes of individualism and consumerism have been steadily gaining ground for over half a century. Modern day parents may want their kids to succeed in school, but their own attitudes and behaviors no longer reflect the old values of externally imposed discipline and unquestioning deference to authority. Meanwhile their view of education remains locked into the only model they have ever known and they push their kids to perform – just as they were expected to perform.

And the kids are not doing well. Even among the 'high achievers' the suicide rates are alarming and constantly rising. Those who manage to claw their way into the boardrooms of the elite will become prime targets for the new breed of psychotherapists and the pill-pushers who promise to bring meaning and happiness back into the over-stuffed world of Lear Jets and waterfront palaces. Meanwhile the pretenders in line beneath them will remain on the relentless treadmill of ambition, dissatisfied with their second-class status and awaiting that elusive opportunity to hit the jackpot before they fall into the cultural catchalls of clinical depression and chronic anxiety. Then we have the multitude of also-rans, ne'er-do-wells, resisters and rebels, all hanging around with their tags and labels waiting for the world to come to them, which of course it never will. According to the science they are supposed to learn, they are all evolving biological organisms - and the system treats them accordingly.

By high school many kids have already given up. Indifferent to the platitudes of their teachers, and disenchanted by the prospects of a meaningless future, they have become conditioned to respond to the bell that signals their transition from English to Chemistry. For them school is no more than a transitory warehouse at best, and a prison at worst. Cooped up together, they turn their frustration on one another, individually and more disturbingly, in gangs. They learn only what they are told to learn, very reluctantly and for the most part, very badly. They can't write or grasp basic mathematics but above all, they can't, or won't, think for themselves – in many cases, they're not even allowed to think. Their interests are not in the classroom but in finding whatever pleasure and gratification can be gleaned from an extra-curricular world that has rejected and betrayed them. The families and communities that once offered places for the aged and young have crumbled in the wake of frenetic materialism,

> *They learn only what they are told to learn, very reluctantly and for the most part, very badly. They can't write or grasp basic mathematics but above all, they can't, or won't, think for themselves – in many cases, they're not even allowed to think.*

and while the old folks are hidden away in geriatric ghettos, the kids are left to learn whatever they can, alone, or from each other. What they seek is not meaning but diversion, an escape from being locked-up for six hours a day, five days a week waiting for the final bell to release them from their drudgery. And who can blame them?

This might seem like a dismal synopsis of state-governed standardized education, but the evidence is painfully apparent – just spend a couple of hours hanging around your local high school. Once the picture becomes clear, you may demand to know who should be held accountable for this squandering of human potential, and when it comes to the education of our children, the options are plentiful. Governments, business corporations, educational authorities, schools, colleges and universities are all convenient targets for our discontent. Such accusations are more a reflection of the problem than a step toward any solution. What we need to understand is that we are all the creators of the systems that govern our daily lives. We have created governments to look after us, corporations to satisfy our material demands and educational authorities to take responsibility for our children and what they should learn – isn't that what we pay our taxes for? Well it simply isn't working, and unless we know what we want and assume responsibility for dealing with the monster we have created, we will always end up in the same disgruntled state. Our kids are in trouble and they need our understanding as never before. If we are to respond rationally and effectively, we had better be clear about the

> *What they seek is not meaning but diversion, an escape from being locked-up for six hours a day, five days a week waiting for the final bell to release them from their drudgery. And who can blame them?*

nature of the difficulty and not simply react to our own discontent by demanding some form of change or taking our frustrations out on the kids themselves. Allow me to make some predictable observations.

If we begin with the assumption that we all come into this world with an inherent curiosity and a fundamental desire to learn, the most basic error becomes immediately obvious: when you compel people to do what they already want to do, they won't want to do it anymore. This isn't some perverse quirk of human nature - it's a basic need of the Self to write its own story. To deal with this annoying tendency, the enforcers are obliged to up the ante by placing the 'target group' under surveillance and subjecting them to a regime of standardized expectations with measurable outcomes. Coercion is then applied through rewards, punishments and threats until an acceptable level of compliance can be attained and managed. Success is measured by the degree to which individuals demonstrate that they act, think and feel according to the beliefs, values and desires, of the prevailing authority. In a society at large this can be a monumental challenge, but if all the subjects are herded together through legal imperatives, the task becomes considerably easier. One time-tested strategy is to create a stratified hierarchy in which the most obedient are given an elevated status and paraded before the lower ranks as symbols of success, the unquestioned and unquestioning products of a system held together by its own dogma. This is as true in totalitarian regimes as it is in the institutions of so-called 'democracies' where young minds are stifled, molded and manipulated from the age of five until they are finally released back into a world constructed through the minds of others.

The Timing Couldn't Be Worse

The time when children are supposed to be sent-off to school - somewhere between ages four and six - conveniently coincides with the period when the child's understanding of the world is already being challenged by thoughts that seem to come from nowhere. It is this growing ability to think that prompts the educators to come-a-knocking. Their interest is not in teaching how to think, but instructing children what to think. But first they must separate the child from what is already known and direct the young mind's attention to what has to be learned. Here there is no place for the sadness of a dying rainbow, the laughter of rain in a crinkled drain pipe, the sweet smell of the parsley patch, and the eerie rumble of monsters in the old junk yard. This is the childish stuff that must be suppressed or ridiculed before the new learning can begin. To move on the learner must come to mistrust both the senses and the imagination in making way for the presentation of the new 'truth.' This isn't a reality to mess around in - it's a cold abstraction that pays little or no attention to personal feelings, hopes or fears. Here the wonder of what 'might be' is replaced by definitive explanations of what 'is.' As the questions become more predictable and the answers more absolute, the malleable and creative young mind is systematically compressed into a cerebral memory bank that sorts information into pre-determined categories called 'knowledge.' The channels that connect the mind to the Self and the Self to the Whole are blocked off and the energy diverted into the neural pathways of dissociated intelligence.

By the second year the system is already beginning to sort out the stars from the also-rans; you don't really need standardized tests to determine which is which. Sitting in grade two classrooms you can easily spot the kids who are less than enthusiastic about the tedious mechanics of the abstract world. In this group you will find the 'daydreamers' drifting back into preferred realities of their own creation. If you look carefully, you will see the 'slow pokes,' those who are only prepared to swallow so much head gruel at one sitting. Unless their appetite improves, they are likely to find themselves drafted into the ranks of the attention-deficit disordered. You will have no difficulty in spotting the 'wild-ones,' those who refuse to have their boundless energy suppressed by authorities that have little or no meaning for them. These are the troublemakers, the ones who must be brought under control if the system is to do its job and to this end, many will be delivered into the hands of the pharmaceutical industry. Then there are the 'hostile ones,' those who have made up their minds to fight back. They know they've been ripped off, even though they may be confused about the precise nature of the crime. In most cases their anger was stirred well before they started school, but now they have a *bona fide* reason and target for their outrage.

Let's Hear It for the Drop-Outs

So there they all sit, the 'daydreamers,' the 'slow-pokes,' the 'wild-ones,' and the 'hostile ones'. They are all resisters; kids who refuse to give themselves up to a brand of learning that pays no heed to their lives on the inside. Yet oddly enough, the system needs them because, within the enlightened hallways of formal education, the success of some can only be recognized through the failure of others. They are the fall guys, the cannon fodder in a calculated assault upon the human spirit. Only when they go too far and threaten the delicate balance of this equation are they suppressed or removed from harm's way.

These are the kids with whom I've spent so much of my professional life. God bless them all. In their own way every one of them knows something is wrong and so do I. We may differ on the 'diagnosis,' but we all understand that they need, and deserve, much better. Far beyond the dismal prospects of academic achievement what they really seek is a sense of belonging, to themselves and within a world that unconditionally affirms their inherent rightness. In his book *The Last Child in the Woods*, published in 2005, Richard Louv identifies their condition as a "separation anxiety disorder." This is not the trite classification based upon the premises of attachment theory and listed in the D.S.M. 1V. What Louv is referring to, is the anxiety that comes from a sense of being disconnected from the natural order – a universal condition that acknowledges every human life as an integral part of the whole. Of course this is not all the fault of the schools, but unless these institutions begin to respond to the developmental needs of children rather than insist the children respond to the needs of the system, the situation can only get worse.

My childhood friend Sammy Reynolds taught me a lot about education and disconnection. Sammy didn't like school and he made no bones about it. His passions were the pigeons he kept in a loft over an old junk shop and his bus trips into the country where he would set them free to find their own way back. Sometimes at weekends and during school breaks, he would wander through the countryside sleeping in the woods and not coming home for days at a time. At the age of fifteen, Sammy was already a loner and he liked it that way. I overheard one of our neighbors describe him as a "troubled young man from a troubled family" but to me he was hero, a kid who lived his own life in his own way.

When he finally agreed to take me on one his 'rambles,' I told my parents I was going on a 'camping trip' with some kids from the youth club and met up with Sammy at the bus depot. He carried his beloved birds, six on this occasion, in a wooden box with holes drilled into the sides. He waited until the other passengers had tossed their bags onto the racks before carefully placing his precious cargo where it was least likely to be disturbed. We sat where he could keep it under constant surveillance. On the outward journey he talked about pigeons – how they all have different personalities and form special relationships with their owners. He told me how one of his birds had been shipped off to Australia and flew past the same boat on its return journey.

On Sammy's instructions, the driver dropped us off on country road where a pastiche of stone-walls and hedgerows followed the contours of a valley and blended into the distant moorlands. It seemed strange to me that two inner-city kids could suddenly find themselves in such a different world and I was struck by how confident my companion seemed to be as he led the way along pathways that were no more than faint indentations through the grass and gorse. After an hour had passed with little said between us, he sat down cross-legged by a trickling stream and placed his bird-box across his knees. "This is the place," he said. "Now we have our freedom, so they should have theirs."

Opening a small trap door at the top, he reached in and took out the first pigeon. Holding it firmly in one hand and gently stroking its head with the other, he began to make a strange gurgling sound with his throat. When the bird gurgled back, he smiled, and raising both hands in the air, he pushed it skyward. "See you soon, Maid Marion," he said quietly as he watched his baby climb toward the clouds, "Don't wait up." Each bird was released with the same delicate ritual; Molly-May, Billy Boston, Little Lilly, Crazy Chris and Princess Patricia were all dispatched with their own message for the trip. I felt like an outsider watching a private ceremony that had never been witnessed before. When it was over Sammy lay on his back with his hands behind his head and stared up at the sky. "They'll all be home before dark," he said. "They don't need to be told. They can only handle so much freedom… just like us." Before leaving, he hid the empty box under a clump of gorse and hooked his knapsack over his shoulder. "We'll pick it up on the way back," he said as we headed up stream, toward the heather and the tree-lined hills beyond.

For the next four days we wandered through mysterious woodlands and across dappled purple moors. With only a blanket each, we took advantage of nature's hospitality, sleeping in hollows and following the trails of unseen creatures toward undetermined destinations. We carried enough food to see us through, but my companion was always on the lookout for berries, roots and plants to enhance our diet of baked beans, pre-cooked sausages and canned rice pudding. "The feast of the forest is fucking fantastic" he said patting his belly and burping his contentment after an evening meal. We never lit fires. "Fires are angry," he said. "I've had enough anger to last me forever. When animals smell fire, they head for the water and so should we." Without Sammy at my side I would have been scared out of my wits, but he always seemed so relaxed and ready to deal with whatever came along. "Are you going to move into the country when you leave school?" I asked one night as the moon cast its aura of eerie light over our mossy nook. "No, I'm a pigeon," he replied. "I like it, but I don't belong here. That mucky old hole in the wall is my home, and yours too."

Only a few months after our five-day 'ramble,' my family moved to another part of the city and I was sent to a school in the new suburbs. Years later in my second term at the university, I came across Sammy standing alone at the bar in a downtown pub. I immediately abandoned my fellow students, and over two or three pints of the landlord's best we shared our stories. Sammy had left school at sixteen and after working for a year with the City Parks Department, he was accepted into the two year

National Park Ranger Training Program and was subsequently given a post in the English Lake District. To me it seemed exactly what he would have wanted so his obvious lack of enthusiasm for his work came as something of a shock. "Things are different when you have to study them," he explained. "I used to go looking for otters because I felt excited being close to them – now I just count them and move on. And the 'sour-dab' leaves that tasted so good with a can of beans - they're *Olaxis Stricta* and stink like cat's piss. Now I walk through the woods like a shipping clerk, checking the inventory and feeling nothing at all." "What about pigeons?" I asked. "Do you still keep pigeons?" "You're talking about *Columbia livia*," he said. "They are townies. As a species they're considered pests because they shit all over the place." "So, no more Maid Marion's eh?" Sammy shook his head and drained his pint. "So what about you?" he asked, "tell me about life at the universitality."

While it didn't occur to me in the pub, I gradually came to understand what Sammy was talking about. I chose to study psychology because I enjoyed being around unruly kids – kids who followed the rules had little to teach me. As a relatively untrained schoolteacher, I wanted to know what each of my students was thinking and feeling as they created their own unique pictures of the world, and I was fascinated by whatever they had to share. Within the classroom, my own life was inextricably bound up in what we were learning, and I loved every minute of it. When I left to work with the 'drop-outs' hanging around the Dock Road, I was even more involved in kid's lives, visiting their homes and insinuating myself into their daily adventures. I was never one of them, but I knew I was part of their world and I always had something to bring to the party. In my early years at the university I was introduced to the principles of psychopathology and theories of juvenile delinquency and my perspectives began to change. I learned about the social conditions that give rise to juvenile crime and decided to become an advocate for social reform. I was introduced to methods for promoting healthy development and pro-social behavior in deviant populations, and committed myself to acquiring the necessary skills.

To focus on my studies, I left my digs on the Dock Road and moved into a University Student Residence where I believed, there would be fewer 'distractions.' Occasionally I would take time out to wander through my old stomping grounds, but it was never the same. I was no longer part of the scene, and I came to see people who had been embedded in my life as empty clichés. Like Sammy's beloved pigeons, they were objects to be identified by their appearance and known through their observable characteristics – my own version of *Columbia livia*. In the pursuit of academic knowledge, I moved away from the lives of kids in order to study them from the outside. This was a conscious decision on my part, although at the time I was not aware of how profoundly this shift would influence so many aspects of my life. In particular, I did not understand that what I had really stepped away from was my Self, my sense of being at the center of my own knowing.

Looking back, I can see how this disconnection had been systematically engineered from the time I first sat in a classroom reciting my number tables. Through twenty years of formal education, I can't remember a time when anyone asked me about my feelings, my life outside the classroom, or my world on the inside. There was one teacher who wanted to know how I "felt" about being in his class, but the question was more about predicting my behavior than artless curiosity. This is a staggering indictment against a system charged with the responsibility for nurturing the development of young minds and teaching them how to create a place for themselves in a complex relational world.

What angers me most is that it really doesn't have to be this way. For me, there is absolutely no reason why introducing children to mathematics, for example, needs be detached from their experiences of everyday life. I'm not talking about measuring the living room carpet or calculating the sum of the angles in the potting shed, although these might be steps in the right direction. My concern is how the inside world of the child is so casually dismissed as being irrelevant, or even contaminating in the learning process.

In junior school, I probably had more feelings in arithmetic classes than in any other segment of the primary curriculum. They weren't the nice feelings good students are supposed to have when they learn something new and receive that coveted gold star. But they were real feelings that had a profound influence on my ability to take in the unfamiliar information. When my performance fell well below the standards set by the gold-star brigade, I lost interest in the competition and began to doubt my ability to recover, no matter how much my teacher and parents shouted encouragement from the sidelines. In high school, my deficiency was painfully apparent, even though I created complex diversions to avoid the scrutiny of the evaluators. I considered myself fortunate to have a math teacher who chose to make both our lives more tolerable by masking the severity of my deficit with what he called "charity marks."

Despite my well-documented progress in other subjects, my secret disability continued to eat away on the inside, creating a generalized sense of incompetence that seeped into all aspects of my life. Whenever I thought about my future, everything I wanted to do seemed to involve mathematics and my aspirations turned into fantasies. Fearing I would not be following my brother into higher education, my parents arranged for me to have individual tutoring, but by this time, the mere sight of a simple equation was enough to bring down the shutters. I didn't want more instruction; I wanted someone to understand my feelings of incompetence and hopelessness. I wanted to be shown that mathematics could be as exciting as Jazz, as challenging as writing an essay, as mysterious as Tibet and as fascinating as the history of Manchester United. But it never happened. Even my personal tutor trotted out the same old stuff in the same old way and I did everything possible to escape from the anxiety of confronting my numerical nemesis. At this point, I disliked school, and my negativity became increasingly apparent in my behavior and subsequently my grades.

There's no doubt in my mind that I would have dropped out at the age of fifteen had it not been for one very special teacher who, for some strange reason sat with me in the 'detention room' and chatted about the similarities between Albert Einstein and Benny Goodman. The following weekend he showed up at the youth club where I was playing in a hotchpotch jazz band for the benefit of kids who couldn't afford to frequent the real dance halls. At his request, I played St. Louis Blues as a clarinet solo and his enthusiastic response triggered an unprecedented round of applause from the characteristically unresponsive gathering. Oddly enough, he never taught any of my classes but he became my link with the school, my reason for doing my homework and a significant mirror of my own worthiness. Thanks to him, I eventually scraped my way into a university – without any demonstrated improvement in my mastery of mathematics.

For the first two years, I carefully steered clear of any classes that might expose my irremediable incompetence, but there was no stepping around the required third-year course in physics. I went to the first lecture, fully prepared to abandon higher education and throw myself at the mercy of the labor market. The class began with film simply titled 'The Universe', and my fears dissolved into awe as the images and music gently massaged my mind and stirred my senses. When the film ended, a figure appeared to walk out of the screen, like a stranger from outer space. "So there you have it ladies and gentlemen," he announced in a soft East Indian accent. "This is your introduction to macro-physics. Take a break and we'll talk about it." Later in the course, he referred to mathematics as 'the music of the spheres' and explained how the same basic principles could be used to enhance our understanding of nature, from the behavior of elementary particles to the expansion of living stars. Without the ability to solve simultaneous equations, I found myself participating in a discussion on the existential implications of 'Planck's constant.' I learned that mathematics was about creating ideas and building models in ways I had never imagined. For the first time in my life I wanted to learn more about this obscure subject and enrolled in a non-credit course in basic calculus. It was a struggle but with help from a devoted friend, I passed with distinction.

Teaching Troubles

Thus far I have avoided identifying the teachers themselves as the front-line agents of educational repression. Most are graduates of the same system and their professional training has demanded an even more intensive commitment to the cause. Although I managed to evade this additional level of assimilation myself, I know only too well how difficult it is to question or subvert a system that has the expressed backing of colleagues, employers and parents. From the challenge of harnessing the boundless energy and curiosity of twenty first-graders, to confrontations with university students who demand an A-plus grade to get into graduate school, educators are obliged to ensure that, above all, the system will prevail. Although they may have considerable latitude in creating their own classroom environment, failure to adhere to this fundamental expectation can have dire and lasting consequences. To be fair, I have come across a number of dedicated and talented educators who bring caring, creativity and compassion into their work. I am also aware of independent organizations that provide 'student-centered' learning approaches, but for most kids the government-operated institutions are all they will ever know, and it is on their behalf that we must advocate for change.

In a previous chapter I appealed to medical practitioners to consider the psychological, developmental and relational aspects of what takes place in the birthing room. My plea to educators is that they open their awareness to all the learning opportunities that become possible when groups of children are brought together in a stimulating and personalized environment. I want them to understand that learning can enrich every moment, rather than become programmed into brains and embalmed in notebooks for future reference. In particular, I urge them to find ways to invite each child's curious and expressive Self into a caring, interactive, and interpersonal learning milieu - an environment that recognizes and respects the contributions of every learner, regardless of where he or she happens to be located on the performance scale. It isn't the brain that craves learning; it's the Self that requires a constant flow of information in order to fulfill its own unique potentials. And no emerging or fulfilled Self is ever superior to, or more worthy than any Other.

> *It isn't the brain that craves learning; it's the Self that requires a constant flow of information in order to fulfill its own unique potentials.*

Of course I would like such ideas to become incorporated into the collective mind-set of instructional bureaucracies, but I have no faith in relying on the guardians of education to make it happen. Such change, if I can call it that, can only come from those who spend their days in face-to-face contact with the educational recipients. There is one essential ingredient that must form the foundation of any movement in this direction. Those who have the privilege of attending to the learning and development needs of children must be prepared to bring their own Selves into the classroom. Any curriculum, however rigid and demanding can be brought to life in the hands of real, live, thinking, feeling and compassionate human beings. And any regime, however draconian, can become relational through leaders who are curious, open, honest, and responsive to those around them. The courage required is not so much about taking up arms against an imagined enemy as about taking the risk to be fully human and fully engaged in whatever might be taking place.

As an untenured and relatively untrained Junior School teacher in the north of England, I delighted in knowing that, once inside the classroom, I was free to set up my lessons in my own way as long as my weekly reports convinced the Head Master I was dutifully following the curriculum. My lesson plans were carefully laid out ahead of time, although they were rarely followed. Invariably one of my students would say or do something that was clearly more interesting than the next step in the sequential learning program and the plan would be shelved – at least temporarily. What I enjoyed most was how, with a little encouragement, the other kids were more than ready to throw their own ideas into the pot, supporting or challenging the validity of the interruption. Sometimes we would set up crazy experiments to test out equally crazy hypotheses and a state of tolerable anarchy would break out. One of my colleagues, a recent product of advanced teacher-training, once collared me in the staff room and demanded to know what all the noise was about. I offered a token apology and explained we were just having some fun. "Save your fun for the playground," he advised. "How do you expect my lot to concentrate on their arithmetic exercises with that racket going on next door? This is a school, not a bloody holiday camp."

To atone for our deviance, we took an hour every Thursday morning to catch up with the curriculum. It was a drag for all of us, but we took our punishment seriously and knuckled down to the task at hand without complaint. It was obvious to us all that sitting in rows made conversation difficult. So each day, immediately after the lunch break, we pushed our desks against the wall and arranged our chairs in a circle, mine included. In my two years of teaching in that particular school, I never came across one pupil who didn't like this arrangement. For the most part our afternoons were spent reading, practicing skills with each other, and at the end of each day, and discussing what we were learning together. According to school policy, we were allowed three 'field trips' each year with monies provided through the 'school fund'. Discussions about where we should go were often long and heated, but in the end, the kids made their own decision. While we sometimes ended up in strange and 'risky' places, I never felt obliged to exercise my unquestionable right of veto.

In case you are inclined to believe I was attempting to implement some unconventional model of education, let me assure you that I was not. I had only flimsiest knowledge of education theory, and almost everything that happened, just happened. Interestingly enough whenever I was called upon to demonstrate my teaching skills to the Head Master or a visiting School Inspector, the desks were always in rows, I stood by the blackboard and the lesson was delivered according to plan. Sensing we were performing for outsiders, the kids played their part in the ritual to perfection – sit up straight, no talking to each other, hand in the air to ask or answer a question, and smile appreciatively when the visitor tells you what a great class you are. Thanks to the dedication of my colleagues in the Kindergarten, we never had to waste our precious learning time on these things.

In odd moments of reflection, I used to think I was encouraging children to manipulate the system and that my pupils would eventually pay a price for our deviance. Yet some years later, while visiting schools in Chairman Mao's China, I watched children sitting in side-by-side desks taking their weekly 'tests.' What struck me was how students who seemed puzzled would look over at their partner's workbook, have a quick word, and blatantly copy down the answer. My fellow delegates were also raising their eyebrows, but the teacher did nothing to intervene. In our subsequent meeting with the Principal, our spokesman shared this observation and wanted to know why such cheating was left unpunished. The Principal, who was also the School Janitor, seemed bemused. "We encourage them to share their knowledge," she explained. Now that's really unconventional.

In those days, all children in Junior High Schools were compelled to take a nation-wide examination shortly after their tenth birthday to determine which secondary school they would attend. Those with the highest marks were admitted to the 'Grammar Schools' where an academically-focused curriculum would prepare them for even higher education on the way to becoming professionals of one sort or another. Those who missed the cut were bundled off into low-status schools with the prospect of either ending up in a trade or taking on one of the more menial jobs that the new professionals would eventually require. It was a cruel and repressive system but at that time it was rarely questioned. A week or so before this examination, our class seemed to lose its vitality. Spontaneity gave way to empty routines and there was little I could do to bring back the life I had come to expect and cherish. On the morning of the trial I stood in the hallway, watching the kids filing into the gymnasium that had been set up like the clerical office of an over-sized insurance company – desks set row upon row and five feet apart. Each of the children in our class came over to make contact, but their eyes had no sparkle and their faces showed little real expression. When the doors finally closed to keep them in and me out, I knew that I despised the system to its very core.

Two or three weeks later, when the results came out, our class exceeded all expectations. Out of twenty-six pupils, fourteen were granted places in Grammar School and six were offered places in specialized trade schools. What made this even more remarkable was that these children were considered to be long shots - working class kids from a working class school in a working class area. When the Head Master called me to his office to offer his congratulations, he told me he had sent an official letter to the authorities requesting that I be given a grant to pursue studies in education at the university. "And I expect you to come back to this school," he said with his hand outstretched. But it was too late. I had already decided that my interest was more with the kids who lived on the wrong side of the educational tracks. I never did tell him how much I had been cheating all along the way.

Almost thirty years later, I was teaching at a Canadian university. My undergraduate classes contained up to a hundred students and were held in lecture theatres for fifty-minute sessions. Clearly there was little opportunity to promote personal interaction, and the only way to have students contact and express themselves was through their out-of-class assignments. Graduate seminars were more conducive to sharing, and I stretched the experiential dimension as far as circumstances would allow. Desiring more student contact at all levels, I moved to a more humble university where the classes were considerably smaller and I made a point of booking rooms that would allow me to create a talking circle. At first the students were uncomfortable with this arrangement, but after one or two classes it was not only accepted but also preferred by most participants. Halfway through the first semester, I grew tired of shifting tables and desks at the beginning and end of every class. It was actually a student who suggested that we leave the circle in place and leave it up to the next class to determine their own seating configuration – a reasonable idea, I thought. But the fallout was completely unexpected. Unbeknownst to me, some faculty members had been questioning my teaching methods and complained to the Academic Dean about having to re-arrange desks and chairs into rows before beginning their lectures. The Dean took the position that it was all a storm in a teacup, and suggested I could avoid further 'unpleasantness' if I would just agree to restore the standard seating after each class. I categorically refused on the grounds that, other than anachronistic tradition, there was nothing in the policy manual to indicate how seating should be arranged for optimal learning. If the university wished to establish such a policy, I would then deal with that dictum. Meanwhile I had to modify their furniture preferences, so there was no reason why they shouldn't have to change mine.

This absurd controversy carved out divisions throughout the Department. Even the office staff felt obliged to take sides, and I found myself being refused secretarial help and starved of basic office supplies. Eventually I had a telephone call from the President of the Faculty Association who threatened "immediate and serious action" if I refused to back down. His wild accusation was that I was deliberately creating tension between the students and their other professors. "I would like you to come to my class and share your opinions with the students," I told him. "Stop playing games," he yapped. "I'm not talking to students; I'm talking to you as a colleague and your President." "Then I expect you to behave accordingly," I said before putting down the phone. A few days later I received a sealed note from the University President's Office. Its message was vague and its tone conciliatory. It concluded: "All things being equal, I would appreciate any action you might take to resolve the apparent differences between you and some of your colleagues." Of course, I took no action but I did take some satisfaction two or three months later when I noted that a number of my colleagues had taken to arranging their classrooms in a circle.

Bureaucratic change may be slow and ponderous, yet it is possible. There are things parents can do to nurture a child's natural curiosity and mitigate some of damage inflicted in the name of education. They might begin by reflecting upon their own school experiences and their attitudes toward education before deciding what they really want for their children. In the final analysis, responsibility for the wellbeing of a child rests with the legal guardians, and short of denying the youngster's access to an acceptable standard of education, they have every right to ensure that the best interests of the child are being served – in or out of school. With this in mind, allow me to suggest a few possible strategies for parents.

What Parents Can Do

1. Choose a school

It's probably not a good idea to burst in on the first day of a grade one class with a list of demands; a progressive, gentle and responsive approach is more likely to be effective. Getting to know something about the school ahead of time is always a good idea. The experiences and opinions of others are certainly helpful, but first-hand impressions are by far the most valuable. Dropping into the quintessential 'office' to reveal your intentions may evoke the offer of an escorted tour, and I can think of no reason why this should not be accepted. Notice whether your guide tends to focus on the programs and facilities or the children and their learning. Then, after the formal information package has been delivered, a more in-depth impression can be obtained by simply loitering with intent, particularly when the bell rings and the pent-up energy pour out into the hallways. Wild exuberance and laughter does not necessarily reflect the joy of learning: more often than not, such behavior is the celebration of a long-awaited freedom. Pay attention to the quiet kids, the ones who seem less inclined to discharge their energy in all directions. Eavesdrop on their conversations and notice if they relate to what is being learned in class. Look for the number of the children who voluntarily remain in the classroom after the bell and notice if the teacher is still involved, or preparing to head out of the door. If, on reflection, you have specific or general concerns about your child being 'educated' in this environment, extend your inquiry to include another visit. If your impressions remain negative, contact the authorities and arrange to review another one of their establishments.

2. Get to know the teacher

Once your child has been 'placed,' take the time to meet with the classroom teacher before the term begins. Ideally, you will come to consider this person as a colleague who will be sharing some of the responsibility for the overall development of your son or daughter. In its impersonal form, the relationship between a parent and a teacher is a legally bound arrangement, and a clarification of mutual expectations can certainly be helpful. There is no substitute for a 'personal' relationship that embodies reciprocal respect, trust and understanding. If the adults share a common understanding of what serves the best interest of the child, the foundation for such collaboration can be established at this initial meeting. If there are significant disagreements where both remain locked into their respective roles, the child will almost certainly pick up on the standoff, and the crucial integration of learning between home and school will be seriously compromised. The responsibility for establishing this connection lies with the adults, although where possible and appropriate, the child should be included in their on-going collaboration. A child who is completely left out of this communication may well come to believe that some form of conspiracy is taking place and respond accordingly.

3. Go back to school

If all goes well at the initial meeting, I strongly recommend you ask permission to 'sit in' with the class occasionally. Notice if the teacher responds to this as an opportunity to collaborate, or as an imposition on his or her territory. If there is obvious resistance or refusal, then the ball is clearly back in your court. Please bear in mind that whatever happens in the classroom is the teacher's professional responsibility, and you are not likely to gain anything by making demands or challenging his or her authority. How your request is handled is simply more information for you to consider as you plan for your child's education. Teachers who are committed and confident in their work will generally welcome the opportunity to involve parents in this way, but there may be exceptional circumstances and these should be noted and carefully considered. If your request is accepted, then follow through with your expressed intention and make arrangements to go back to the school.

I realize what I'm suggesting may be a challenge for many parents. To some degree most of us felt powerless in school and the prospect of returning as a collaborator may well evoke feelings of resistance, apprehension and even fear. Even if you don't anticipate such reactions, sitting at a desk in a grade one class can quickly bring the unexpected to the surface. The familiar sights, sounds and smells of your school days can arouse the senses and give rise to a multitude of feelings, thoughts and attitudes. Pleasant or unpleasant, the task is to recognize these experiences as vestiges of the past: you are not enrolled in the class and you are there for a different reason. Paradoxical as it might sound, by acknowledging and bracketing off these feelings and thoughts, you will be better able to place yourself in the position of being a child in that class with those children and with that teacher, at that moment in time. Your senses will then be free to take in the quality of life and learning in the classroom. In particular you will have the opportunity to decide for yourself whether the children, including your child, are actively involved or sleeping partners in their own learning. As a bonus, a teacher who has welcomed you into the classroom should also welcome your impressions as collaborative feedback, and your relationship will be strengthened.

4. Establish a home-school connection

I've already mentioned the importance of creating a link between classroom learning and what takes place in the home. This is a connection that can only be effectively consummated through the experience of the child. In this regard the token question "How was school today, Honey?" and the perfunctory reply "We learned all about frogs today – see ya later, Mom," fall far short of the mark. Your interest in your child's classroom learning validates the youngster's natural curiosity and makes it possible for you to elaborate and deepen this learning through everyday experiences. It is not your role to teach the curriculum or make up for what you consider to be the deficiencies. If you have a solid relationship with the teacher these are matters to be addressed, and hopefully resolved, at your next meeting. Reciprocally, you should also be prepared to consider what the teacher has to say about his or her perspective on the connection between the classroom and the home. Just as teachers can become defensive about their performance in the classroom, parents can over-react to anything they perceive to be a criticism of their family or their parenting. Potentially this can be dangerous territory and underscores the need for a mutually respectful personal relationship. A shared commitment to work together can usually transcend such difficulties and regular meetings, preferably with the child present, are immensely valuable. Encouraging the young student to speak up in meetings and in the classroom is one of the important steps toward self-directed learning.

It's easy for any parent to become lost and confused within the labyrinth of a public education system, and attempting to influence the workings of such obdurate bureaucracies can seem like a monumental challenge – which of course, it is. Recognizing and respecting the points of accountability not only saves time and energy, but also increases the likelihood of being heard. In this regard, the simple rule that the teacher is in charge of the classroom and the Principal is in charge of the school is always worth remembering. If parents wish to have an active voice in the overall operation of a school, no forum has more potential options than a well-organized and supported Parent-Teacher Association.

5. Participate in the P.T.A.

Getting involved in the P.T.A. is a step most parents can take. Having worked with a number of these organizations, I remain enthusiastic about their potential and saddened by their general ineffectiveness. All too often they end up as little more than insignificant or convenient adjuncts to a system that traditionally resists any form of outside interference. In my experience, P.T.A.'s committed to influencing life and learning within the school struggle to articulate their role clearly and can quickly become bogged down in their own internal politics. When it comes to the philosophical and methodological principles of education, they either defer to the experts or take adversarial positions that prompt the system to close ranks. Yet these are the very issues that should be out in the open, generating dialogue between the professionals who provide formal education and the parents whose children are the unwary recipients. Time and again, I have seen 'new' theories and approaches being introduced into educational programs with parents having little or nothing to say about the matter. Meanwhile, the active members of the P.T.A. are busy organizing a bottle drive to purchase paintings for the school foyer. In this way the system preserves its exclusive status, and the broader debate that should be taking place on critical matters of education is effectively snuffed out at the grass roots level. For me, the real tragedy is what children learn when they see their adult caretakers backing off from confronting the authorities that prescribe and govern our lives. Individually, this is homage to obedience and, collectively, the most fundamental principles of democracy are effectively bushwhacked.

Whenever I talk to parents about these things, I try to remain practical and positive, but it isn't easy. My own experiences are always there to remind me that, despite all the challenges of the past, some accommodating, some radical, our formal systems of education have remained essentially unmoved; if anything, they have become even more resilient and repressive. The only real difference is that kids are finally beginning to question their legitimacy and see school for what it is – an uncompromising assault on the human spirit. The predictable response of the 'leviathan' has been to dig in further, spurred on by the 'back to basics' brigade who call for more discipline, more punishment, more authority, more control and more standardized tests. These things, they say, should be established in the early grades before the rot sets in.

Much as I believe we all have a responsibility to shape the kind of formal education our children receive, I also fear that an open dialogue on education would reveal that the public school systems are doing exactly what we want them to do. It may well be that the vast majority of parents are quite happy to have their kids taken off their hands for five days a week and subjected to a regime that pits child against child in a senseless contest between success and failure. Perhaps they don't really want their children to experience the excitement of following their own curiosity. Maybe they're afraid that if their children came to know and understand their rightful place on this planet, they would rise up in anger – better to punish them for their deviance than reward them for their insight. Whatever the questions and whatever the answers, the dialogue needs to take place. If the outcome serves to support the status quo, then so be it. At least we will be left with a system that reflects the beliefs of the majority and for which that majority can be held responsible.

Parents Still Have Some Options

One ominous indicator is that the voices that once cried out for change are no longer to be heard. Through the 1960's, 70's, 80's and 90's, the writings of A. S. Neil (*Summerhill*); John Holt (*How Children Fail*); John Taylor Gatto (*Dumbing Us Down*); William Glasser (*Schools Without Failure*); George Leonard (*Education and Ecstasy*); Charles Silberman (*Crisis in the Classroom*); Herbert Kohl (*The Open Classroom*), and many others, not only urged us to put the learner at the centre of the learning, but encouraged educators to create new possibilities and initiate alternative programs. Sadly this is no longer part of the mosaic. Somehow the machine has managed to roll on, flattening out the ground and crushing the tender shoots that once gave promise of a different kind of future. Despite its relentless determination, children are still children and their potential to become all that they are, to explore the frontiers of our humanity, still simmers within them. The question is, do we have the will and the courage to set them free?

> *Somehow the machine has managed to roll on, flattening out the ground and crushing the tender shoots that once gave promise of a different kind of future ... do we have the will and the courage to set them free?*

Despite my obvious pessimism, I continue to believe that parents do have the power to influence the educational system and even pull the plug, if they have a reason and the will to do so. Whenever they move in this direction, I am with them all the way. Short of embarking upon a collective crusade, they still have individual options outside the formal labyrinth. For some, private and independent schools offer a range of alternative programs and philosophies. But scholarships and subsidies aside the fees are generally high and, for many parents, prohibitive. Alternatives like the Montessori and Waldorf schools are usually less expensive and within the reach of parents who have more modest resources available for their child's education. Yet, simply because a school operates independently doesn't necessarily mean it does things differently. Many parents are prepared to pay large sums of money to send their kids to educational boot camps where the competition is intensified and the consequences for failure and non-compliance are even devastating.

Home as an Option to School

At the other end of the spectrum are those parents who choose to opt out of the formal education system completely and teach their own children – at home. Reaching its peak of popularity in the 1980's, home schooling was enthusiastically supported by a prominent group of professional 'drop-outs' led by American educator John Holt. Disillusioned by the obvious resistance of the establishment to any form of external influence, they argued that children learn best through direct interaction with the real world within the context of everyday life. The uncompromising nature of their defection from the system that once fostered their ambitions and paid their salaries is tersely expressed in Holt's declaration: "What is most important and valuable about the home as a base for children's growth in the world is not that it is a better school than schools, but that it isn't school at all" (*Teach Your Own* p. 213). In response to those who argued that parents were not qualified to teach and could never attain the standards expected within the formal system, the renegades insisted that the evidence was to the contrary. In his book *Dumbing Us Down; The Hidden Curriculum of Compulsory School*, published in 1992, *John Taylor Gatto* wrote:

The home schooling movement has quietly grown to a size where one and a half million young people are being educated entirely by their own parents; last month the education press reported the amazing news that children schooled at home seem to be five or even ten years ahead of their formally trained peers in their ability to think. (p. 26)

While home schooling remains a viable option for parents who are willing and able to assume this responsibility, its popularity has been steadily declining over recent years. Part of the reason may be that schools are now geared toward providing career-packaged education and parents are concerned that their kids will not receive the specialized knowledge and skills demanded by the corporate employers. At the same time, the number of families in which both parents are engaged in regular employment has been increasing dramatically. The irony is that many of these parents are working to save money for their children's 'education.' I have no idea what it would take to change this mindset, or the system it serves to perpetuate. It seems we have become so accustomed to the separation of parenting and education that we cannot imagine them to be integrated aspects of the same developmental process. By the same token, the experts who assume the role of educators are unable or unwilling to accept that learning takes place within the subjective experience of the learner. In most areas the curriculum and standards for home schooling are established and controlled by local educational authorities according to their own 'in-house' criteria. When all is said and done, it still remains the responsibility of every parent to decide what form of 'education' his or her child should receive.

Considering all the above, I know that if was back in their shoes, I would do everything possible to avoid committing my child to the public school system. My reasons are many but the root of my concerns are exquisitely expressed as follows:

He always wanted to say things. But no one understood.

He always wanted to explain things. But no one cared

So he drew

Sometimes he would just draw and it wasn't anything. He wanted to carve it in stone or write it in the sky

He would lie out on the grass and look up at the sky and it would be only him and the sky and the things inside that needed saying.

And it was after that, that he drew the picture. It was beautiful. He kept it under his pillow and would let no one see it.

And he would look at it every night and think about it. And when it was dark, and his eyes were closed, he could still see it. And it was all of him, and he loved it.

When he started school he brought it with him. Not to show any one but just to have it with him like a friend.

It was funny about school.

He sat in a square, brown desk like all the other square, brown desks and he thought it should be red.

And his room was a square, brown room, like all the other rooms.

And it was tight, and closed, and stiff.

He hated to hold the pencil and the chalk, with his arm stiff and his feet flat on the floor, stiff, with the teacher watching and watching.

And then he had to write numbers. And they weren't anything. They were worse than the letters that could be something if you put them together And the numbers were tight and square and negated the whole thing.

The teacher came and spoke to him. She told him to wear a tie like all the other boys. He said he didn't like them and she said it didn't matter.

After that they drew. And he drew all yellow and it was the way he felt about the morning. And it was beautiful.

The teacher came and smiled at him. "What's this?" she said. "Why don't you draw something like Ken's drawing? Isn't that beautiful?"

It was all questions.

After that his mother bought him a tie and he always drew airplanes and rocket ships like everyone else.

And he threw the old picture away.

And when he lay out alone looking at the sky, it was big and blue and all of everything, and he wasn't anymore.

He was square inside and brown, and his hands were stiff, and he was like any one else. And the thing inside him that needed saying didn't need saying anymore.

It had stopped pushing. It was crushed. Stiff.

Like everything else.

-Anonymous

CHAPTER SEVEN

Adolescence Ain't What it Used to Be

Since the end of the Second World War, compulsory schooling in western societies has created the context in which the transition through puberty into adulthood has become a sub cultural phenomenon – a defined category within the social matrix. Responding to the pressures of consumerism and empowered by commercial opportunism and media attention, yesterday's confused kids have become today's expressive, demanding and defiant teenagers. As Marcel Danesi notes in his book *Cool: The Signs and Meanings of Adolescence*, published in 1998, "without a high school environment to sustain it teenager-hood as we know it would disappear" (p xi). In his analysis of the semiotics of adolescence in North America, Danesi shows how specific language forms reflect a discrete and complex sub culture with its own symbolic, attitudinal and behavioral characteristics. Within this system, the much sought after 'ego-identity,' described by psychologist Erik Erickson in the 1950's, has been molded into a distinctive persona designed to impress peers and carve out a place within the broader reference group.

On the surface, all this might appear to support the traditional notion of adolescence as a transitory period when rapid physical and psychological growth interact with social conditions to create characteristic patterns of

For most kids the modern teenage sub culture is not regarded as a preparation for life in the adult world.

adjustment along the final stretch into adulthood and social assimilation. From this perspective schools have provided kids with an opportunity to share this developmental challenge. Closeted together behind red brick walls, they have created their own collective response to the uncertainty and anxiety of establishing a place for themselves in the world as independent and responsible contributors. From here we might be led to believe that in general, today's teenagers are simply following in our footsteps, experimenting with their independence before setting out on their careers and forming families of their own.

But this, I believe, would be a fundamental mistake. For most kids the modern teenage sub culture is not regarded as a preparation for life in the adult world. It does not contain the traditional rites of passage common in less complex societies, and its expressed values and aspirations often appear as oppositional to those within the mainstream culture. The well-worn idea that teenage rebellion is a normal and necessary step toward adult independence cannot define or account for what has taken place. We are talking about a well-established and diversified segment of society that has become a permanent fixture and potentially, an agent for change. In order to consider the implications, it might be helpful to take a look at how and why this cultural phenomenon came into being. My primary purpose in offering this brief idiosyncratic review is to challenge the common belief that teenagers are still hanging about in the wings waiting to assume their role on the adult stage.

Enter the Global Teenager

In the 1950's, high school kids in North America were actively engaged in transforming the in-school peer group into a national, and even international, sphere of influence. Recognizing these youngsters had money to spend, this phenomenon was promoted and choreographed by media and commercial interests always on the look out for new markets. The popular teenage culture symbolized and incorporated most of the aspirations and fantasies generally associated with adolescence – the quest for identity and belonging, the blossoming of sexuality, the assurance of rightness and identification with role models and heroes. All were addressed through slick marketing and image management to generate a highly energized and idealized teenage way of life. Fads and fashions were promoted and paraded before millions of receptive consumers, while the music industry created a plethora of romantic balladeers to croon over the virtues of teenage love and Saturday night cruising. Even as Frankie Avalon and Paul Anka tugged at tender emotions, there were clear signs that a darker aspect of the teenage psyche was waiting to be unleashed and exploited – one that would be far less acceptable to the ears of the moral authorities. Elvis Presley, with his pelvic thrusts and derisive sneer, set the early alarm bells ringing while rock and roll moved from the innocence of Bill Haley's Rock Around the Clock to Jerry Lee Lewis's ambiguous "Great Balls of Fire". As Danesi points out, actors like James Dean and characters like Holden Caufield in J.D. Salinger's iconic work *The Catcher in the Rye*, revealed an undercurrent of angst lying beneath the fun-filled lives of the "Happy Days" generation. Meanwhile in the United Kingdom, John Osborne's play *Look Back in Anger,* dramatized a movement in which a new breed of artists set out to express the disenchantment of modern youth with the world they are obliged to inherit.

The first cohort of graduates from the new teenage sub culture delivered a fascinating and unexpected message. Rather than accommodate to the materialistic values in which they were nurtured, or adopt the cynicism and hostility of the dissenters, large numbers of these young people chose to 'follow their bliss' by breaking away - or 'dropping out' - from the mainstream. Their banners of 'Love' and 'Peace' were presented as antidotes for a society obsessed with consumerism, competition, achievement and confrontation. In true adolescent fashion, their cause was to break free from the old shackles of security and express their independence, not through rebellion, but more through the strategies of passive resistance personified by Mahatma Ghandi.

As you might expect their understanding of how the world worked was naïve, their values were idealistic and predictably, their broad aspirations turned out to be unattainable. But as a *bona fide* social movement, they had taken the first step toward assuming ownership of their own destiny. Both the moral authorities and commercial opportunists lost their influence and power because they failed to recognize one basic developmental need at the core of the emerging sub culture. The essential quest of the 'me' generation was neither moralistic nor materialistic - it was spiritual; a search for meaning beyond the prescriptions and routines of everyday life. In this area the mainstream had little or nothing to offer, and the kids were free to explore and create their own meanings in their own way – and this they did with commendable dedication.

The essential quest of the 'me' generation was neither moralistic nor materialistic - it was spiritual; a search for meaning beyond the prescriptions and routines of everyday life.

To a large extent, their symbols and lifestyles arose from their own grassroots creativity, and nowhere was this more apparent than in the progression of their music through the 1960's. In 1964 the Beatles released their first album *Please Please Me* – a compilation of trite pop singles that had created the commercial backdrop for 'Beatlemania'. Three years later they produced *Sergeant Pepper's Lonely Hearts Club Band*, and the shift was staggering. With its psychedelic tapestry and sophisticated recording techniques, each track on this album used satirical and abstract imagery to reveal a counter-culture that was so far removed from conventional wisdom that it could never be effectively assimilated into the mainstream. In Britain's most respected conservative newspaper The Times, celebrated columnist Kenneth Tynan referred to the release of Sgt. Pepper as "a decisive moment in the history of civilization." His adulation was not for the artistry of the product but for its unpretentious dismantling of consensual reality. Predictably the reactionaries dismissed such praise, claiming Sgt. Pepper to be no more than a drug induced distortion – a clear confirmation that kids were drifting away from reality and needed to be brought back into line.

There could be no turning back, and from the Mecca of Haight Ashbury in San Francisco to London's Hyde Park and Moscow's Red Square, young people discovered a common ground – an opportunity to share and celebrate their uniqueness, and in a spiritual way, their togetherness. Of course the moguls of the media and the music industry moved in on the action, but this time they were not the ones calling the shots. For this brief and magical moment in time, 'flower-power' was in, and in so many ways its impact influenced an entire generation.

From Revolution to Rapprochement?

At first blush, it might be easy to dismiss the psychedelic sixties as a fleeting diversion from the true course of history. It is 'true' that many of the youthful freedom seekers eventually ended up trading in their beads and bandanas for business suits and brief cases. This transition was dramatically exemplified when Harvey Newton, the leader of the radical Black Panther movement, gave it all up to market his own brand of B.B.Q sauce, but that's not the point. The point is that young people had become a defined reference group with the collective ability to communicate their ideals within their own communities, across this continent and throughout the world. Even more to the point the concept of the teenage sub culture as a shared and lived in reality came into being just as we moved into the communication age. From that point on it was clear that kids would continue to have their say one way or another. The media and the messages may not have remained true to the idealism of the 1960's, but teenage sub cultures have continued to make their presence felt even in the most repressive and draconian circumstances.

In North America we have seen many twists and turns in the evolution of youthful sub cultural activity over the past fifty years. The fracas at Woodstock, armed confrontations at Kent State University, protests against the Vietnam War, Black Power, and the rise of Muslim theology were early signs of a growing unrest among young people. As with all social movements, the youth sub culture became diversified, each faction responding to its own specific interests and conditions. This diversification is reflected in particular dress and behavior codes, but above all it is the musical forms that have most clearly expressed the relationship of each group to the dominant culture. Romantic ballads, lyrical protest songs and good time rock and roll lacked the specificity required to say what really needed to be said. While their basic elements were retained, they became differentiated into Soft Rock, Disco, Hard Rock, Punk Rock, Heavy Metal, Hip-Hop, Reggae, and Rap - each having its own meaning and making its own statement to the world. By the same token, smoking pot or dropping acid has given way to a miscellany of drug options -including heroin, crack and crystal-meth - that serve to characterize particular sub cultural factions within the whole. The question as to whether we can still talk about a teenage sub culture as a common reference group is certainly debatable, but I believe that within the broader context, the movement that began fifty years ago is a reality that needs to be acknowledged and, above all, heard and understood.

No Risk, No Freedom

Given the emergence of the adolescent sub-culture, we need to recognize that these young people have created a world that is related to, yet different from, the mainstream; a lived in reality with its own distinctive past, present and future. The transition from puberty into adulthood can no longer be viewed as a well-trodden pathway from confusion and uncertainty to clarity and purpose in an orderly world.

We are now at the point where confusion and uncertainty are entrenched in most mainstream cultures across this planet, and none of the self-righteous 'democracies' can claim to have a clear and purposeful platform for the future. This is not an orderly world – far from it. At some level we all know our future on this planet cannot be protected by the promises of the power seekers, preserved by the platitudes of the peacemakers or procured by the prescriptions of the prophets. Rather than confront our fears we have chosen to live in denial, desperately clinging to the illusions of the 'good life.' We are still obsessed with the insatiable demands of the ego and will take up arms against anyone, or anything that stands in our way. In case you don't recognize it, this is the stuff of adolescence. At the core we are as ˙confused and fearful as the kids who continue to drift around in transitional space searching for the elixir that will bring meaning and substance into their unfulfilled lives. Their sub cultures may offer some immunization from the prospects that loom before them, but as the creators of that reality, the onus is upon us to step beyond the adolescent mould by taking responsibility for our actions.

We are still obsessed with the insatiable demands of the ego and will take up arms against anyone, or anything that stands in our way ... we are as confused and fearful as the kids who continue to drift around in transitional space searching for the elixir that will bring meaning and substance into their unfulfilled lives.

This isn't about frantically scurrying around to find solutions to our current ecological, social, economic and political problems for the sake of future generations. These are simply reflections of our fear driven delusions, and nothing will change until we recognize that we are the problem – each and every one of us. Recycling our garbage, voting for the 'right' party, boycotting supermarkets and donating to worthwhile causes, may give us a sense that we are doing our part to bring about change. As valuable as these actions may be, they should not distract us from the greatest challenge of all – finding the courage to acknowledge the root of our fears and changing our way of being with ourselves, each other and all that surrounds us. Only by exploring and revealing the core of our humanness will we offer our children a legacy of lasting value. We can no longer urge them to play out their lives according to our scripts and use their dependency to enforce their compliance. We need to recognize that, whatever their age or their place on the developmental continuum, their world is not the same as ours and learn to value whatever they bring to the party.

This applies as much to the inscrutable seventeen-year-old as it does to the gurgling infant. When we can acknowledge our own agendas and move beyond rejection or confrontation, the world of the teenager offers remarkable insight into our own camouflaged dreams and fantasies; not as they were, but as they are. Once we realize that what they seek is essentially no different from what we seek, conflict and coercion give way to curiosity, understanding and caring. Regardless of what has gone before, the passageways of communication are never permanently blocked and the more it takes to ease them open, the more incredible the discoveries and the more profound the feelings of mutuality. I categorically reject the common belief that what we call 'adolescence' is a time when kids naturally close out their parents and turn to their peers. The movement toward individuation and independence is an incremental progression and in some way, every shift changes the nature of the parent-child relationship. There may be glitches here and there but in the long run, the transition usually works to the benefit of both parties.

Where breakdowns occur the seeds of discontent are more likely to be found in the actions and attitudes of the parents than the unacceptable aspirations of the renegades. By this time, conscious and caring parents who have accommodated their child's developmental shifts from total dependence through

> *Once we realize that what they seek is essentially no different from what we seek, conflict and coercion give way to curiosity, understanding and caring.*

healthy narcissism and rapprochement, will understand what's taking place and want to be fully available to offer support and encouragement through this critical period. Up to this point, every step along the way has called for insight, caring and at times, setting limits, but always with the underlying assumption that Mom and Dad have the final say. Now parents must learn how to release the last vestiges of their power with the same sensitivity and understanding. To make matters even more difficult, they must learn how to operate from the assumption that their irrational teenager is responsible for his or her own decisions, whether they the parents, believe it or not. Above all, they must learn how to do all this without sacrificing the integrity of their own personal aspirations, their own values and their own way of life. In close family relationships, learning is a mutual affair.

What parents need to understand is that the timorous Self requires an identity, a persona, to define its place in the world beyond the parameters of the family. For many kids, the teenage sub culture is the testing ground, and its distinctive values, attitudes and modes of behavior are essential to the cause. Certainly there are risks involved, but the kids who really find themselves in trouble are those who for whatever reason, have decided that anything is better than what they leave behind and burn the proverbial bridges. Difficult as it may be for anxious parents to believe, this is a time when their children need them to be 'there' – not as supervisors or service providers, but as pillars of security and integrity who can be relied upon when the going gets tough and the boundaries between fantasy and reality dissolve into chaos.

Free the Parent, Free the Child

In my experience, youngsters who have the most difficulty making this move toward independence have parents whose own sense of individuation and freedom is sadly lacking or glaringly incomplete. They need their kids far more than their kids need them. This isn't something that suddenly appears when a son or daughter passes beyond family picnics and hot chocolate at bedtime. As long as parental authority is considered to be legitimate and effective, anxieties and resentments can be kept under wraps. Once the quest for freedom is set in motion, the bindings begin to unravel and the hostilities begin. Parents who remain caught up in their own agendas may try to retain their power by attempting to suppress the unruly spirit. Some manage to achieve this, but the developmental damage, individually and relationally, is far deeper and more lasting than any wounds inflicted through open warfare. Whatever the circumstances, rebellion and repression are not part of nature's design. Within the continuum, parents who have moved beyond their own adolescence to establish an individuated sense of Self will understand the struggle, take a breath and grant the necessary freedom - just as they did when their toddlers took their first precarious steps or locked the bathroom door.

I'm not suggesting that parenting a teenager should be a piece of cake. The fact is I've never talked with any parents who could honestly say this was a period of uninterrupted harmony. It is, and always will be, a pivotal episode in the evolution of the parent-child relationship in which the parties are equally challenged to learn how to redefine their roles and relate to each other at another level. This doesn't mean they should learn how to become 'best friends.' Their relationship will always be like no other, and however close and individuated they might become, the parent will always be the parent, the daughter will always be the daughter and the son will always be the son. Nor am I implying that this transitional period cannot be successfully negotiated unless all the tensions of the past have been resolved. There will always be 'stuff' to deal with, but that's what makes the learning so meaningful and mutual. I have worked with many parents who, on reflection, reported that the struggles to live with a defiant teenager prompted them to take a closer look at themselves, and they were amazed by what they discovered. In some cases they began with the familiar "where did we go wrong?" lament but found they were able to move beyond the fixation of blame to recognize that they did their best at the time and there are always new possibilities to explore. In effect they initiated another step in their own development of Self and in so doing, became more curious about the experiences of others, including their unappreciative teenager.

Their relationship will always be like no other, and however close and individuated they might become, the parent will always be the parent, the daughter will always be the daughter and the son will always be the son.

Having spent so much of my life working with unruly kids, I'm well aware of the frustrations that can arise when confronted with hostility or passive resistance. Over time I've come to appreciate the virtue of patience, while constantly suspending my own agendas and replacing them with artless curiosity. Time and again I've struggled with the risks of non-intervention and in hindsight, there were times when perhaps I should have stepped in earlier. Risk is an essential factor in the equation and managing anxiety part of the solution. More often than not, what seemed like a tragedy in the short term, turned out to be a pivotal learning event for at least one of us. Thankfully I'm still learning and my beliefs continue to be delightfully unstable. But there is one conclusion that has remained firm for many years – there isn't a teenager on this planet who, given the opportunity, doesn't want to be seen and heard by an open, honest and compassionate 'elder' who has learned how to live beyond what others want and think. Attachment to peers and immersion in a sub culture may be the order of the day, but deep down all kids know that this space is transitory and need an anchor point in the world they are destined to inherit. Meanwhile, the world they inhabit is as real and challenging as the one that lies ahead, and its legitimacy needs to be affirmed from the outside. When viewed with open curiosity, rather than predetermined judgments or patronizing tolerance, it offers a fascinating glimpse of the human psyche that cannot be obtained from any other source. Getting to know and understand this world through the minds and emotions of those who participate is a privilege I will always appreciate.

There isn't a teenager on this planet who, given the opportunity, doesn't want to be seen and heard by an open, honest and compassionate 'elder' who has learned how to live beyond what others want and think.

The Search for the Grail

At the beginning of this book I stated that it was not my intention to offer cookbook recipes for being with children, and I remain committed to this stance. The time when both parent and child must come to terms with whatever went before and learn how to relate to each other as separate yet connected Selves creates its own challenges and possibilities. Even those parents who have been solid enough in their own sense of Self to allow increasing degrees of freedom along the way may find their time tested approaches are no longer effective. Looking at it from another point of view, youngsters who have been relatively successful in moving along the developmental continuum can easily lose their way in negotiating the maze of conflicting values and divided loyalties that lay between them and their quest for identity. With this in mind I would like to offer some guiding principles for your consideration. While these are primarily intended for the benefit of adults, they are not offered as parenting prescriptions but as possibilities that can promote the self-development of both parties. In the broadest sense, I believe them to be essential ingredients in any relationship that aspires to promote a meeting of Selves.

1. Learn to stand back from the action and consider what is taking place

Like any other social system, the family is structured according to differential individual responsibilities and defined codes of behavior. Within this framework, children are generally expected to assume increasing levels of responsibility while learning the behaviors that are acceptable to the parents and society in general. Of course there are consequences for failing to live up to these expectations. Without this structure, kids would have no way of defining themselves or acquiring the skills necessary to create their own pathway in the world. Ideally most of the roles and rules remain responsive to new information and changing circumstances, but there are always 'bottom lines' - non-negotiable commandments that form the bedrock of the family's values and beliefs, such as "Thou shalt not kill thy younger brother for being an insufferable reptile." The significant feature of these rules and regulations is that they are essentially impersonal; they do not belong to any one individual but are adopted into the policy manual of the family as a whole. In themselves, they do not create relationships but provide the context in which each family member can feel safe and protected. For this, there can be absolutely no doubt that ultimate responsibility for articulating and enforcing these conditions rests with the parents.

But when a restless young insurgent sets out to claim the status and rights we call 'adulthood,' even the most open and responsive system should be ready for a shock. Whatever has been stifled in the past may rise to the surface, catching everybody off guard and producing a reactionary backlash from those on the receiving end. In such cases, parents may attempt to re-affirm the traditional roles and enforce the old rules, but the gods are not on their side. Driven by destiny, the crusaders are hell-bent on carving out a new role, and rules that have not been accepted and internalized by this point become ready made banners for the crusade. They know their cause is noble and their ambitions pose no threat to anyone who already has a clear and secure a place in the realm. What they seek can never be taken from or given by another; it is something they must create for themselves even in the face of powerful resistance - a new identity, a reconstructed version of the 'me.' In essence this is a recapitulation of the entitlement and unabashed narcissism that appeared over a decade before, and whatever was left from that first leg of the journey will be back to seek resolution. Now the process is considerably more complex and penetrating. It is complex because cognitive development and emotional differentiation have created a highly intricate world of perceptions, abstractions and aspirations. It is penetrating because those same abilities can be turned either inward or outward. Simply stated, the Self now has the capacity to be its own witness – to observe itself in action and examine its own internal experiences. With all of this going on, it's hardly surprising that the young person may at times appear moody, detached and self-absorbed. The good news is that parents who have continued along their own developmental pathway will be even better equipped to understand and respond accordingly this time around –it's all part of growing up together.

To define its place in the social order, the new 'me' requires an insignia, a recognizable identity that represents its unique qualities and affirms the dignity and rightness of the bearer. The symbols may be challenging or celebratory, but either way the purpose is to create a safe location from which the authentic Self can find expression and set the course of its own destiny. To this end, the evolving 'me' takes its instructions from the invincible 'I" while negotiating with the external authority for its legitimacy in the scheme of things. There may be periods of impasse or outbursts of hostility, but as long as the external authorities remain open and responsive, the negotiations will proceed and eventually all rights and privileges of the realm will be bestowed upon the newcomer. The empowered Self is free to continue its journey.

If confronted by constant rancor and resistance however, the quest for identity degenerates into a battle for survival. On the inside, the task becomes the protection of the 'I' while, on the outside, attack is often chosen as the best form of defense. In this process the 'I' steps out of the arena in much the same way as a nation abandons its humanity when it decides to go to war. The longer the hostilities persist, the more the insurgents become identified by their oppositional attitudes and insubordinate behaviors within the family and beyond. Unknown for who they really are, they become locked into their postured identities and deviant roles. With no access to their own inherent sense of 'rightness,' they are left to construct a self-view based upon the judgments of others; to become outlaws, rebels, druggies, drop-outs and the like. Some will continue to fight and others will choose to abandon their cause, but unless something happens to change the course of events, an unfulfilled and restless Self will remain locked away in its solitary stronghold. This, more than anything you might read in a psychology text or psychiatric manual, defines my work with kids for most of my professional life.

Noble metaphors aside, I have never taken the position that the answer lies in granting unconditional access to the status of adulthood – whatever that term happens to mean in any given society. If there were no expectations to be met and no obligations to be fulfilled, there would be nothing of value to strive for. The inherent cause of the Self is always toward higher levels of awareness, expression and responsibility, and these are not attained through passive compliance to the existing order. On the other hand if there is nothing to come up against, no defined structure to confront the ego and no resistance to test the mettle of the adventurer, the Self will never develop the strength it requires to sustain its journey. This is not the time for significant adults to defend or abandon their own beliefs, values or lifestyles. Rather, it is a time to stand firm, yet responsive, while the young seeker discovers his or her own point of entry into the system and makes the necessary arrangements.

What really needs to change is the nature of the relationship. Within the developmental continuum, the power that once held everything together is gradually replaced by the 'personal', a more equitable and responsive arrangement in which the 'I' of each participant comes to know and respect the 'I' of the other. In making this shift the adult says, "I have done my best to protect and guide you over the years and in return, I have expected you to follow my instructions and live according to my beliefs and values. But the time has come for you to take charge of your own life, and my hope is that you will always consider whatever I've been able to

Now I want you to know me as I really am – not just as the person who changed your diapers, put food on the table and told you to be home before nine, but as a fellow traveler with my own history, my own fears, my own hopes and my own feelings.

offer. Now I want you to know me as I really am – not just as the person who changed your diapers, put food on the table and told you to be home before nine, but as a fellow traveler with my own history, my own fears, my own hopes and my own feelings. Whenever you are ready to hear these things, I will be ready to share them. And, as you move toward creating your own life in your own way, I would like to know more about your journey. What you choose to tell me may not be what I want to hear, but I will do my utmost to understand. If I have judgments or suggestions, I will share them with you, but only with your permission. And, whatever happens along the way, I want you to know that I love you and I have confidence that you will become the person you truly are."

This may sound like a rather wordy good parent message, and that's precisely what it is. It is different from those energetic messages that shape the early development of the Self since it is primarily conveyed in words and actions and received through complex thoughts, reflections and feelings. The focus is not so much on the emerging Self of the receiver as on the relationship between two separate Selves and expresses the simple desire to know and be known by, another human being. But the energetic foundations must also be present. If the words carry the authentic feelings of the sender, they can be taken in by the Other at all levels. In effect, this message is a standing invitation for the 'I' of the recipient to remain open to the outside world, whatever the circumstances. This is the essence of adult relationships that are not bound by rules and roles but negotiated through the personal boundaries of each authentic Self.

2. Work toward replacing roles and rules with personal boundaries

When people talk about their "boundaries," they are usually concerned with protecting themselves from the physical, emotional and psychological intrusions of others. This is not what I mean by the term. Here I am referring to the parameters that define and contain the Self in all its energetic, subjective and expressive forms. Without such boundaries there can be no identifiable Self and in any given relationship, it would be impossible to determine where one person ends and the other begins. In our work with couples we have often encountered this confused state of enmeshment, and you may recall the case of Laura where the Self of a daughter became merged with that of her mother. A boundary affirms the presence of a unique and separate human being, and its function is more about reaching out to explore new possibilities than protecting the status quo. Most critically, the boundary belongs to the Self, and each person must take responsibility for preserving its integrity and effectiveness. When two Selves engage at the 'contact boundary,' the possibility of relationship begins.

If the core of the human Self is energetic, then its most essential boundaries must also be experienced and expressed energetically. This might be conceptualized as a unique life force that generates a distinctive energy field vibrating from the inside and extending beyond the skin into the outside world. There's nothing mystical about this notion. Even the standard instruments of science are able to detect a human presence in an energy field, and each presence radiates its own distinctive resonance. As the most sensitive and sophisticated of all sensors, we are much better equipped to appreciate the qualities of that presence. As an example, think of all the times you've been aware that somebody is around, even without visual or auditory confirmation. In particular, consider those situations where your senses tell you that you are being watched, when the energy of another person is focused in your direction. If your senses are open and receptive, you will also pick up the quality of that energy, including that person's attitude and intentions.

The energetic boundaries of the Self are flexible, constantly moving in and out in response to whatever is happening in the broader field. When the Self is secure, the boundaries are exploratory, moving out into the world and seeking connection. When the Self is unsure, the boundaries are drawn in, moving with caution and vigilance. If the external world is experienced as being threatening, the Self will seek protection by replacing its flexible boundaries with rigid defenses or walls. Children who grow up in a hostile and abusive world direct their self-energy into the construction of walls, and however much they learn to cope with their circumstances, the liberation of the Self will never take place unless these defenses are replaced by contact-seeking boundaries. Inviting and encouraging children to make this transformation has taken up a significant portion of my professional life.

If the Self remains open yet contained within its own parameters, its energetic core gradually assimilates thoughts and emotions to form the workings of a unique 'complex' system. At the same time, the senses become increasingly attuned to differential stimuli from the outside and this information is accommodated into the system, generating what we call 'self-awareness.' For this to occur, the boundary must remain sensitive and responsive to the outside world while ensuring that the integrity of the emerging Self is preserved. Such a Self will learn to move freely in the world, constantly adjusting the space it requires as circumstances change. By expanding and contracting their own energy field, people with effective boundaries can remain present and engaged while choosing the degree to which the Self will participate in any given situation. At the core energetic level, the need to make such adjustments is not recognized through thoughts but through feelings; sensations located in the body. If you would like to experience this directly, you could invite someone to collaborate with you in the following exercise.

> *Begin by sitting on the floor with your partner fifteen to twenty feet away. Take a deep breath and notice what this contact between you feels like in your body. Now invite the other person to move closer, two or three feet at a time and pausing at each stage. Notice what happens in your body as that person approaches. Be aware of your breathing. Continue until he or she is almost touching. After checking in with your body, ask your partner to move back to the original distance. Once you feel settled, take a piece of chalk (or yarn, string, or something similar) and make a circle around yourself. Take a breath and imagine yourself filling that space. If the circle seems too large or too small, make whatever adjustments you wish – paying attention to what your body has to say. When you feel comfortable with the space you have created, make a statement of your boundary to the other person, something like "This is my space; please stay out of it unless I invite you in." Notice what happens in your body as you say this. Now ask your partner to begin moving toward you in the same way as before until he or she reaches the edge of your boundary. Notice if your space now seems too small or too large and make whatever changes you wish. At this point you have a boundary and the other person does not. How does that feel? Now invite your partner to draw his or her own circle and make a boundary statement. What do you feel in your body? Is your experience of the contact between you the same as before the circles were drawn, or different? Are your boundaries distant, touching or overlapping? Now*

reverse roles and allow your partner to have the experience of creating the initial boundary while you make the journey back and forth. When the sequence is complete, take the time to share your personal experiences – you might be surprised what you can learn from each other.

In this exercise, most people discover that having a boundary makes them feel more secure and actually enhances the quality of personal contact. For people who fear abandonment, drawing a circle and making a clear statement may give rise to feelings of isolation, while those who have experienced significant personal inundation may create reinforced circles with overly assertive boundary statements. Either way, the key is to stay with the feelings, to experience them fully and come to know their purpose and their origin. Whatever happens, this simple little exercise can provide a wealth of information for the dedicated observer of the Self.

Energetically speaking, personal boundaries are experienced as a felt sense in the body. While this is most readily apparent in the arena of physical space, the same principle applies at all levels of subjective experience. Boundaries contain the emotions and an integrated sense of Self implies that a person's feelings can be experienced to the full and either expressed or contained as a matter of choice. Emotional space can be created, vacated and violated, just like physical space. Ignoring or overpowering another person's feelings has essentially the same effect as walking away from a friend in need or barging into an occupied bathroom. By the same token, the cognitive aspects of the Self can be overridden by the verbal tirades or intellectual intensity of a dominating other. The implications are that the more the Self becomes known and expressed, the more it is capable of processing internal and external information and the more refined its boundary becomes.

With this in mind, it's not difficult to understand the importance of learning to create and sustain effective boundaries during that critical period of transition between adolescence and adulthood. As the powerful and protective role of the parent begins to soften, the youngster enters an exciting, creative and at times, fearful period in the evolution of Self. Establishing personal boundaries is an integral part of this process and is essential for the development of self-responsibility. Boundaries are created from the inside out, and learning the fundamentals usually involves considerable experimentation; constructing walls, creating rigid partitions and sometimes having no boundaries whatsoever. This learning takes place through direct interaction with significant others, and is most profoundly influenced by those who are able and willing to bring themselves to the contact boundary. Since this is unlikely to take place within a teenage peer group, the family becomes by far the most effective arena for such learning to occur. When a parent is able to say, "I am not telling you to live your life my way, but whatever choices you make, I will not allow you to impose them on my way of being in the world," a clear and informative boundary statement has been made. When that same parent is also able to say, "And I will respect your freedom to do likewise," the foundations of the relationship are affirmed and the learning can begin.

As the powerful and protective role of the parent begins to soften, the youngster enters an exciting, creative and at times, fearful period in the evolution of Self.

Boundaries are revelations of the Self in action and, as in any relationship the learning is mutual. Given this understanding, a parent can become a living example of how firm, yet sensitive, boundaries serve to define and preserve the integrity of the Self. Through everyday events and exchanges, the adult can demonstrate the curiosity, empathy and skills required to understand and respond to another person's boundaries without loss of Self. This requires openness and honesty, always with a gentle invitation for the other person to engage in the same way – to meet at the contact boundary. There are always risks to be taken, hurts to be acknowledged and long standing defenses to be dissolved, but when the exchanges become truly reciprocal the energy flows freely back and forth, the rigid patterns become flexible and the relationship moves from the pragmatic to the personal. There is no simple prescription that will bring this about, but the following story might help.

BOUNDARIES IN RESIDENTIAL TREATMENT

As Senior Therapist at a large treatment center, I became concerned about the quality of life in a residential unit for ten adolescent boys. Simply stated, these guys were deemed to require firm and consistent measures to control their acting out behaviors. The psychologist in charge had designed a highly structured program of predictable and 'natural' consequences, but felt he had to up the ante in the face of escalating resistance, aggression and violence. In the struggle for control, the tensions between the residents and staff created an atmosphere in which personal relationships had become virtually impossible. These are the classical conditions of what we call 'institutionalization' – the impersonal application of rules and the implementation of repetitive daily routines. To break up this pattern we transferred five of the younger boys to another residence and moved in five adolescent girls. It was a radical decision that caused considerable consternation both on and off the campus, but that's another story.

The short-term impact was certainly dramatic, but it wasn't long before the honeymoon was over and the boys began to re-assert themselves, individually and collectively. The daily incident reports showed a steady increase in aggressive acting-out episodes, and as concerns for personal safety became paramount, the staff began to resort to their familiar controlling strategies. When the girls initiated a meeting and demanded they be returned to their original residence, there was a general consensus that the experiment had been a failure, but I was able to convince the managing psychologist that this might be a wonderful opportunity to conduct some creative research.

With the assistance of the research department, we began by converting the incident reports into data sheets and tracked the patterns of aggressive behaviors over a three-week period. During this time, we manipulated schedules to make it possible for the staff to gather each day while the residents were in school. Together we examined the house rules currently in place and from an extensive list, identified six behaviors that would be met with an immediate and known consequence. The rest were to be put on hold for the duration of the experiment. We then set up training sessions in 'working with boundaries' involving all members of the staff, from the housekeeper to the program manager. Using experiential exercises like the one described above, participants were encouraged to explore and express their own boundaries in a safe and controlled environment. To modify the conventional mindset, we introduced the proposition that most rule violations were actually boundary violations and the most effective response was not to punish, but to teach. This involved considerable discussion and practice but by the end of the third week, the unobtrusive monitoring systems were in place and we were all set to go.

The first two or three days of the experiment were noticeably chaotic and the data confirmed an increase in emotional outbursts and acting-out behaviors, well above the established 'baseline'. Things settled down much quicker than we had anticipated and by the end of that week, the climate in the residence was remarkably calm. From direct observations and analysis of the data, the most critical factor seemed to be that staff members were becoming increasingly confident in responding to behavior from the place of their own boundaries rather than the rulebook. During the second week, they began to intervene in disputes between the residents with a clear statement that boundary violations were simply unacceptable and would be taken as learning opportunities. Physical violence (one of the six bottom line offences) still carried the consequence of immediate removal to a 'quiet room,' but as soon as the offender declared himself or herself to be ready, a counselor would be available to work through the boundary issues, often involving the individual who had been on the receiving end of the violence. On re-entry into the group the aggressor joined the evening 'talk-back' session to share his or her learning with the group as a whole and receive whatever feedback the others had to offer.

On the Saturday of the second week, the residents participated in a six-hour experiential workshop similar to the one offered to the staff three weeks earlier. By this time, the term 'boundary' was in common usage and the basic principles were generally understood. It was one of the most exciting and satisfying workshops I have ever had the privilege to lead. With one exception – a young fellow who stoically refused to have any part of it – the kids and staff talked as never before. Among the residents it was obvious that the girls led the way while the boys cautiously allowed their feelings to be known. There was no doubt in my mind that the girls would not be returning to their residence on the other side of the campus.

When the experimental period was over and the data analyzed, even the hard-nosed voyeurs in the research department were impressed with the 'outcomes'. The incidence of aggressive acting-out behaviors had plunged well below the baseline and 'quiet room' confinements had been reduced significantly, while staff satisfaction and resident surveys were overwhelmingly positive. Our research colleagues were quick to point out that some of this might have been due to the "Hawthorne Effect" - a short-term response to any sudden change in conditions; the rest of us were all convinced it was more than that. Having reviewed these findings, residents and staff gathered together and issued a joint manifesto in which they announced their intention to retain personal boundaries as a fundamental principle within the program. After thirty years, I still treasure this document; it stands as confirmation that young people can make responsible choices on their own behalf - even if they happen to be living in a residential treatment centre.

Before going any further on the topic of boundaries, I want to take a brief leap from the logical to the paradoxical. In the above discussion, I have argued that the parameters of the human Self are essential in defining a person's existence in the relational world and, at the psychological level, I continue to believe this to be the case. I have also suggested that the boundaries of an individuated Self are primarily moving toward connection rather than separation - an affirmation of our relatedness. But if you happen to believe as I do, that in the realm of universal consciousness, there are no such divisions, then at some point the lines we have drawn around our Selves must eventually disappear. The logic in this belief is that if our Self-awareness makes it possible for us to delineate our existence, then the essence of who we really are must be able to step outside this place and the Self we have come to know, even energetically, is a fabrication - an illusion if you like. In returning to the universal order, this illusion must be removed at some point. Whether or not this can take place while we are contained within the physicality of the human form is a question for the mystics and may even be answered by future generations. If you wish to examine this matter further, you could do no better than read Ken Wilber's book *No Boundary*, published in 1985.

My only reason for raising this issue is to acknowledge that, throughout this book my focus has been on the psychological realm rather than the universal or transcendental. At this level, the creation of personal boundaries is central to the developmental process we call 'individuation.' Along this continuum, the eventual dissolving of boundaries requires a dismantling of the Self-as-known, but this is not possible if no Self has been created in the first place. Could it be that this process of construction and deconstruction is an essential ingredient in our contribution to the universal order? God knows, I've come across many seekers who claim to have found the pathway to universal consciousness without having to scramble through the rubble of the everyday life-world but, with the odd exception, I have found their presence to be fleeting, insubstantial and distinctly ungrounded. For most of us who struggle 'to be' on this planet, the process of self-construction remains as a life-long challenge with momentary glimpses of what might lie beyond. But without the journey, the destination is also an illusion. At some point in our evolution, all this might change, but meanwhile I will return to my concerns with the kids who must learn how to live within the realities we impose upon them.

3. Use boundaries as a foundation for self-responsibility

Effective boundaries are a necessary condition for self-responsibility. People with a clear sense of their own boundaries are able to engage fully in relationships without losing their Selves along the way. They claim their own physical space, identify and embrace their own feelings, say their real yes's and no's and make decisions appropriate to their own needs while remaining sensitive to the needs of others. On the inside, they are uniquely themselves, taking ownership of their experiences, regardless of the actions and attitudes of others. They are aware of their own body feelings, in touch with their own intuition and can remain fully present in the here and now.

Self-responsible action affirms the belief that we all have the power to make choices in creating our own lives – and vice versa. By this I mean that self-responsibility and a belief in self-determination feed off each other. During the period we call adolescence, this item of self-determination is very much on the agenda. The question is not only "Who am I," but also, "How much am I able to take charge of my own life and make any changes I wish in myself, my relationships and my circumstances?" The way a young person deals with these existential questions is not always apparent from his or her presentation to the world, but the internal dialogue is inescapable.

A CASE IN POINT

Murray was a young fellow who came to see me under rather unusual circumstances. His father made the appointment because he wanted his eighteen-year-old son to take over the family business, but the lad's expressed enthusiasm was belied by his lethargic performance in the workplace. The family doctor had used the term 'bi-polar' and offered to make a psychiatric referral, but both parents refused to believe that their son had some form of mental illness. I found him to be a bright and articulate young man who appeared to be quite at ease and self-assured during our first session. Psychological tests indicated a well above average I.Q. and a relatively high level of self-esteem, but these were offset by a 'locus of control' measure that raised some interesting questions. As a general rule people who feel good about themselves also believe in their ability to act on their own behalf, but whenever Murray tried to make independent decisions, his confidence evaporated. At our third meeting, during a guided imagery session, Murray's presented self suddenly fragmented through a torrent of sobs and tears. Supervising others in his father's business became a nightmare as his subordinates gleefully took advantage of his hesitancy. Not wishing to be seen as a failure by his father, he did everything he could to sidestep his supervisory responsibilities, but his sense of ineptitude was constantly reinforced by these evasions.

During the course of our sessions, Murray began to see how his confidence had always been drawn from his father's approval and his decisions were almost always made with this in mind. He was unable to remember any time in his life when he actually made a decision that was for him and him alone. Tearfully he lamented, "The truth is, I don't even know what's in my own best interests and I probably never have." As long as Dad's support was available he could sustain a positive self-image, but with little sense of his own volition, he was ill prepared to impose his own authority on the workers in the factory. Being the owner's son was his only source of power, but even this quickly evaporated through the constant challenges coming from those he was supposed to supervise. Beyond this arena Murray struggled to maintain the air of confidence he had always presented to the world but on the inside, his assurance was now being eroded day by day, and he felt alone and abandoned.

At a time in his life when nature would have him testing out his efficacy in the world, Murray was heading in the opposite direction, in retreat. This unhappy state of affairs was being held together by an enduring belief that he was not, and never could be, in charge of his life. From experience, he had come to the conclusion that whatever happened to him, including his own actions and feelings, was determined by forces beyond his control, and his best way to cope was to follow the signs. When I pointed out that this was actually a choice he had made, it was clear from his response that he didn't really understand what I was talking about. Whenever I invited him to consider what it might be like if he identified what he really wanted and set out to get it, his momentary excitement was quickly quashed by his entrenched self-limiting belief system. When we took a look at his developmental history, it was clear he had never experienced that narcissistic phase of infancy and because he lived off the approval of others, he felt no urge to rebel during his early adolescent years. Now, thanks to the experience in his father's factory, the voice of the authentic Self was finally being heard, though not yet understood.

Working with Murray involved taking him back to re-experience and repair the early developmental interruptions. Helping him to make contact with his authentic Self and create effective boundaries laid the foundation from which he could begin to make choices on his own behalf and take ownership for the consequences. Unlike many of the teenagers who have found their way into my life, Murray was ready to work, and step-by-step his obvious delight in making decisions on his own behalf urged him to review the evidence that had always supported his restrictive beliefs. The acid test came when he told his father that he really didn't want to take over the family business and had decided to use his grandmother's inheritance to study photography. The old man was gob smacked, but seeing the determination in his son's eyes, he eventually relinquished his own agenda and gave his blessing. Later, when I ran into father at a local bookstore, he accused me of using my influence to sabotage his business. I think… I hope… he was joking.

4. Recognize the importance of making choices

When it comes to making choices, the issue of whether a particular decision is good, appropriate, moral, or even responsible, is not the central issue. The simple act of making a conscious choice expresses the power of the Self to influence internal experiences and external events. The actual choices will, of course, be guided by the nature of the Self, which in its authentic form, expresses the essence of our humanness. Beyond this the possibilities and options are limited only by an individual's personal belief system. Murray for example, may have made conscious choices, but his self-limiting beliefs made him a prisoner of his circumstances. Oblivious to his own inner voice, his decisions were usually based upon what the world expected and to this cause he handed over his own destiny.

Despite the evidence provided by Bruce Lipton in *The Biology of Belief*, most of us assume that some things are unchangeable and impose limitations on ourselves before even trying. My old teacher and mentor Will Schutz used to invite his workshop participants to consider the following hypothesis: I choose my own life, and I always have. I choose my behavior, my feelings, my thoughts, my illnesses, my body, my reactions and my spontaneity. His intention was not to impose an alternative belief system but to invite people to re-examine their own beliefs and identify their limiting assumptions. As the workshop progressed however, the vast majority of participants became aware of their old assumptions and began to explore new possibilities. In particular they were able to recognize the multitude of choices they were already making, with or without awareness. His radical proposition was that awareness is itself a choice and whatever thoughts and feelings we don't

Awareness is itself a choice and whatever thoughts and feelings we don't want to deal with, we choose to deposit in the unconscious

want to deal with, we choose to deposit in the unconscious - the implication being that the unconscious is of our own making and what we choose to put there we can also choose to bring back into awareness. In Murray's case, this might partly explain why when he began to question his self-limiting beliefs, the hurts and stifled aspirations of his childhood came flooding to the surface.

5. Find the courage to tell the truth

And ye shall know the truth,
and the truth shall make you free.
(John 8:32)

The period known as 'adolescence' is typically a time of confusion and doubt. Beneath the pursuit of what's 'cool' lies a much deeper search for what's real, substantial and reliable. Behind the quest for the ego-identity, the questions "who am I?" and its essential corollary "who are you?" become dynamically juxtaposed in the ongoing search for Self. The superficial reality of 'cool' may be constructed from postured images, shifting values and pleasing illusions, but the ongoing evolution of the Self requires nothing less than the 'truth.' On the inside, access to that truth is available through the senses and generally manifested in the body. Whatever machinations the mind might manufacture, the body never lies – although it can be temporarily tricked or numbed out by drugs or medication. On the outside the Self relies upon the availability of incoming information, particularly from the Selves of significant others. The quantity and quality of this information is profoundly influential in determining how the Self comes to recognize its potential and find its location in the scheme of things.

> *Whatever machinations the mind might manufacture, the body never lies – although it can be temporarily tricked or numbed out by drugs or medication.*

In its essence the Self is incorruptible and cannot be deceived, even when the mirrors it encounters are intrusive and distorted. When one person attempts to deceive another, both Selves are equally compromised and the 'lie' becomes locked into their relationship. Energy is diverted into unproductive channels, and whatever the mind might do to justify the strategy, such duplicity can never stand alone as a momentary lapse. Like a virus in a computer it remains as a threat to the integrity of the whole until the necessary steps are taken to remove it from the system. We all know how the most innocuous little lie, motivated by the most noble of intentions, can create an increasingly complex network of intrigue that continues to consume energy and leave the parties feeling drained, confused, anxious, depressed and distant. This is an unsatisfactory state of affairs in any significant relationship, but when it arises between a parent and a teenage son or daughter, the developmental implications are particularly far reaching.

The most innocuous little lie, motivated by the most noble of intentions, can create an increasingly complex network of intrigue that continues to consume energy and leave the parties feeling drained, confused, anxious, depressed and distant.

Obviously my use of the term 'truth' is not drawn from some notion of abstract or objective reality. I am talking about the reality of my own experience, my understanding of 'what is,' perceived through my senses and contained in my thoughts, my feelings and every cell in my body. This is not the truth - it is my truth. When I pursue this truth I become my own internal witness, carefully noting my observations while constantly reviewing the data in the light of new evidence. When I speak this truth I express the integrity of my being without condition. When I deny or withhold this truth from others or myself, my body tightens, my mind distorts and my relationships become contrived.

Intuitively, we all know this but our agendas so often override our wisdom. This applies as much to parenting and teaching it does to pursuing our careers or getting the best deal on our new car. Our culture not only condones but also promotes strategic lying and withholding. We use words like 'tact', 'diplomacy', and 'manners' to euphemize our fabrications, and when we want moral justification, we can always claim that the truth is not in the other person's best interests – we don't want to hurt their feelings after all. In the broader context, we have come to expect and accept that politicians, corporations and salespeople will feed us 'disinformation' to promote their own interests; that's just the way the world works. Is there any wonder kids who are struggling to discover their own truth come to mistrust the information they receive from the outside?

If you were one of them, what value would you place on someone who could be relied upon to tell the truth with awareness and honesty? By the term 'awareness' I am referring to the degree to which a person actually draws from the truth of his or her inner experience. The unconscious is full of things we don't wish to know about ourselves, and the more we stash in there, the less we know and the less we have to share with others. Truth without awareness is shallow and insubstantial. 'Honesty' simply refers to our willingness to self-disclose, but here again without awareness all the sincerity in the world will not compensate for the lack of substance. On the other hand, awareness without honesty is a deliberate withholding and creates the void in which confusion, manipulation and intrigue can run rampant.

Levels of Truth

Based upon the above principles, the inimitable Will Schutz devised a schema that identified five levels of truth. Although this was primarily intended as a device for improving communication in the workplace, it is equally applicable to all significant relationships, and I have found it to be extremely effective in working with teenagers and their parents. It is a fine example of the many insightful contributions Will made to our understanding of human relationships. In providing the following synopsis, I know he would graciously accept my interpretation of his work.

Level Zero: "From You I Withhold". This refers to situations in which I feel something important but choose not to express it. This accounts for the overwhelming proportion of all my feelings.

Level One: "You are ..." Here I am willing to express my thoughts and feelings but the focus is always on the other person. Simply offering an opinion or judgment is a step toward the truth – even if it is derogatory. Calling a lethargic teenager a "useless lay-about" might not enhance the relationship but, at least, something is being communicated.

Level Two: "Toward you I feel ..." This introduces new information into the relationship – my feeling state. The focus shifts from the other person to how I feel within myself, even if my stance remains distant and critical. Telling the same teenager, "I've come to dislike you and want you out of my house" is certainly a more personal statement, although the message may not be graciously received.

Level Three: "Because ..." Now I offer more information about the basis of my feelings. My reasons may be rational or irrational, depending on my level of awareness, but I am prepared to explain and justify my stance. At this level I might say, "I work hard to keep this family going and all you do is hang about waiting to be serviced."

Level Four: "From you I sense ..." This opens up the possibility that my feelings about the other are based upon perceptions that may or not be accurate. I may search for clarification but I continue to hold the other responsible for my experience and can easily see myself as a victim. From this level I might tell my recalcitrant teenager, "You don't have any respect for me as your father. You think I've let you down because I can't afford to pay for you to go to... "

Level Five: "I fear I am ..." When I relate at this level, I recognize my tendency to project my unwanted thoughts and feelings about myself onto others. With this awareness, I can come to know my truth, and I am free to share this with whomever I wish. Should this happen to be my son or daughter, I might take the risk to say, "Sometimes I think I could have been a better parent. I wanted you to have the very best, but there's only so much I can do on my salary. On the other hand, I know I've always done my best for you and my family – that's just the way it is."

Neither Will Schutz nor myself is suggesting we should always tell the truth, the whole truth and nothing but the truth, regardless of the circumstances. I certainly wouldn't tell all to someone I believed would use this information to hurt me, or others. Nor would I share my deepest feelings with a person I just met at the Pub, any more than I would talk to a seven year old about the intricacies of my sex life. I accept the principle that telling the truth is the best policy, but there are always circumstances that call for caution and containment. Much of this has to do with personal boundaries. I am always cautious about sharing my truth with people who are unable to understand and appreciate the difference between my experience and theirs. Similarly I am not prepared to sacrifice my boundaries by allowing my thoughts and feelings to leak out whenever the opportunity presents itself.

Pragmatically, if I tried to do this, I would spend my entire life spilling the beans to all and sundry and there would be no time left get on with day-to-day tasks or pursue my own interests in my own way.

As a guiding principle, telling the truth is always the preferred option, but there are special relationships in which it might be considered an objective to work toward. People seeking intimacy through self-revelation, for example, will continue to dig deeper into their personal truths in order to know themselves and become known to the other without conditions. This isn't about 'letting it all hang out'; on the contrary, it is a project that demands considerable dedication and discipline. Personally, I believe this to be the greatest and most rewarding challenge on the human journey although I know very few people who actually walk this pathway. To a lesser degree, people who share a common cause cannot afford to have their working energy diverted into wasteful strategies of deception and ego-management. As Will Schutz so clearly demonstrated in his work with business corporations, learning to tell the truth can have a profound impact on job performance, productivity and personal satisfaction.

I believe the relationship between a parent and a teenager is also a special case that should embody the same principle. This presents particular challenges however, since such relationships are bound up in their own unique histories and contain elements that are essentially non-negotiable – a parent will always be a parent, even when functional roles are reversed. Much will depend on how truthful a parent has been through the earlier childhood years and the degree to which the youngster has been able to hear and understand whatever has been shared. Ideally this would be a developmental process in which the content and complexity of information provided by the adult remains attuned to the youngster's level of emotional, cognitive and social development. This being so, moving through adolescence would simply require a seamless incremental shift in the quality and quantity of truth available to a young Self as it seeks to establish its place in the adult world. On the other side, an attentive parent would gladly take the opportunity to explore his or her personal truth about relinquishing authority, while gaining more insight into the fascinating truths of a modern teenager.

Such theoretical ideals are never fully attainable. Even in the most committed and caring human relationships, emotional blocks, subtle deflections, unconscious evasions and slippages in attunement are all grist for the mill. Extrapolating the concept of 'good-enough parenting,' such imperfections actually offer the most significant opportunities for both parties to learn more about Self and enhance the quality of their relationship. By illuminating the interruptions of the past, the adolescent experience offers a renewed opportunity for personal reflection and growth, and the more serious the interruptions turn out to be, the greater the potential for change. What matters most is the courage to look and the commitment to hang in, but once again the onus is upon the parent to take the initiative. When he or she decides to give up, close down or seek refuge in the rationalization "You are now free to run your own life, so good luck," the loss occurs on both sides. There is work to be done and a well-intended parent might be tempted to settle for the old cliché, "what's happened is water under the bridge, so let's make a new start." Unless the shadows of the past are acknowledged and confronted, they will continue to find their way into whatever is taking place in the present. These are the sole property of the adult, and only the proprietor has the power to bring them into the light. Of course all youngsters have shadows of their own, but when their time comes, the courage to seek them out will be fortified by having a parent who has shown the way.

This doesn't mean parents should suddenly abandon their established roles and begin to divulge their innermost feelings and darkest secrets to their kids – heaven forbid. All I'm suggesting is that supporting youngsters through adolescence offers a timely opportunity for adults to delve a little deeper into truth; in the service of their own growth and development. Whatever they chose to share with others is a matter of personal choice, and given their awareness of their own boundaries any decision is the right decision. In considering what to share with their children, the following additional questions might be considered:

- Is this something I simply want my son/daughter to know about me or do I have some other agenda?

- Will my son/daughter be able to hear and understand what I have to say?

- Will my son/daughter understand that this is about me and not about him/her?

- In what ways will sharing this information contribute to my son/daughter's own development of Self?

- In what ways will the sharing of this information enhance our relationship?

Such questions don't need to compromise the truth principle, although they can certainly be used as rationalizations for undisclosed and manipulative strategies of communication. It's worth remembering that a commitment to telling the truth does not imply a commitment to complete self-disclosure. "I'm not willing to share this information with you now" can be an honest statement that will be readily accepted by anyone who understands and respects personal boundaries. If the youngster keeps pushing, the most helpful response is not to slam the door but to remain open and engaged. For example, this might be an appropriate moment to examine how it feels when another person chooses not to be revealing. In this way the parent can demonstrate the difference between establishing a boundary and building a wall – wonderful learning for both and for their relationship.

This is what I consider to be the stuff of 'conscious parenting', but it doesn't come easily. In fact a parent who chooses to explore and reflect upon the truth, past and present, may experience as much confusion and anxiety as a teenager seeking a new identity in a separate location. The difference is that the youngster is intent on creating a new version of reality while the work of the adult is more reflective and to some degree, remedial. During this time it's perfectly reasonable for a sixteen year old to expect support and guidance from a parent, but this doesn't work the other way around.

When two parents are able to support each other through this transitional phase, the potential benefits are both personal and interpersonal. This isn't about standing together and presenting a common front to their disobedient kids. On the contrary, this is an opportunity for them to communicate their truths and come to know one another at a deeper level. At the same time, teenagers who witness this form of personal exchange are invited to look beyond the roles to see their parents as separate and unique human beings actively engaged in creating their own relationship. Developmentally speaking, the timing is immaculate and I can think of no greater gift for a young person who is wondering what it really means to be an adult in a relational world. If a parent has no supportive partner, or has difficulties exploring personal truth, a professional therapist might be considered. If so, it's important to keep in mind that this is a personal decision to move to a deeper level of awareness and not an indication that something is wrong and needs to be fixed. It should also be clear that the work is about the parent's own experience and not about a third party – partner or child. Therapists who are not able to understand this position should be avoided.

Freedom through the Family

It is with some trepidation that I now turn my attention to the family. To paraphrase a familiar T.V. announcement, "The following material may be offensive to some readers; personal discretion is advised." My basic stance is that the role-based and culturally defined family we have come to know so well is completely incapable of sustaining us through any shift toward higher levels of consciousness and relatedness. In the West, we have already pushed this configuration to its limits, and the evidence of its demise is everywhere. Those who cry out for its immediate resurrection seem to believe that our social and moral decline has been somehow caused by our abandonment of 'traditional family values' in favor of self-indulgent liberalism. My own version of the causal train runs in the opposite direction. I believe our ongoing search for meaning and connection is our most central developmental task, and traditional family values along with the values that support nationalism, materialism and religious fundamentalism, are counter to this cause. When I consider the sorry state of this planet, I am more inclined to attribute our predicament to our blind attachment to these archaic beliefs and practices than to any form of self-promoting liberalism. So like any confused adolescent, I move cautiously around in the labyrinth, playing with illusions and hoping to find the way out. I refuse to believe that all will be well if I retrace my steps and return to home base.

The role-based and culturally defined family we have come to know so well is completely incapable of sustaining us through any shift toward higher levels of consciousness and relatedness.

It's not that I've given up on the family as the primary vehicle for procreation, nurturance and socialization – although there are alternatives. Call me old fashioned, but I still believe children are best cared for by parents who share a loving relationship. I have no problem with the idea that every family has a right to its own boundaries and identity. We need to understand that the 'traditional' family was never designed to nurture individual Selves and promote relationships among them. Its essential purpose was to provide social and economic security, and its basic structure was designed around specific roles within a power-based hierarchy. For generations it served this purpose well, but by the beginning of the twentieth century, the functional integrity of this unit was beginning to erode. Women claimed their right to vote, men began to realize there was more to life than putting bread on the table and educated children were being invited to question the old adage that father knows best. And the questions kept coming. The moral authorities established by governments to keep the multitudes in check (most notably the Church) could do little to stop the erosion. Even the revered state of Holy Matrimony became an optional contract, subject to renegotiation and conveniently dissolved if one party decides to throw in the towel.

Yet somehow, the old values of authority, ownership and property rights have continued to prevail; protected by the State and embodied in the laws of the land. When this faceless authority falters and we are confronted with the prospect of settling our squabbles person-to-person, we cry out for justice and demand satisfaction. We want the system to be fixed by whoever is deemed to be accountable. The authority has no Soul, and however many social workers we toss into the mix, human emotions and developmental needs will never be incorporated into the system. So when parents decide to split and the law steps in, all the reports and expert testimony in the world will never override the fundamental value that children are chattel to be allocated as part of the settlement rather than being acknowledged as separate beings in their own right.

The problem is not that we have rejected the old values: the real problem is that we are afraid to give them up. Turning back is not an option. Our future rests in our willingness to look closely at what is and draw from the innermost resources of the human spirit to create what we really want. Given my belief that we are all Selves in search of connection, the basic ingredients of the human family – loving and committed adults caring for welcomed and respected children – can be blended into a design that would nurture and support this developmental imperative. But what might such a family look like and what would we have to do to make it work?

The Vision of Virginia Satir

Like everything else in the universal order, the family functions as a system; a configuration of relationships that becomes an entity beyond the sum of its parts. In the 1960's and 70's this perspective was taken up by a handful of adventurous psychotherapists, most notably Virginia Satir. Having watched this immensely talented and creative woman work on a number of occasions, I became convinced that she had taken us behind the scenes to witness the most basic struggle of the human spirit to survive and become known in a world of relentless expectations and rigid prescriptions.

With everyone sitting in a circle, Virginia would gently invite each member of the family in turn to bring his or her thoughts and feelings into the moment, using her indomitable presence to confront anyone who attempted to use the occasion to speak for, or judge, another. Then, with delicate skill and sensitivity, she would draw the family into direct person-to-person interaction, intervening only to seek clarity or ensure that everybody was heard. Her obvious respect for each individual, for his or her position in the family and for the family as a whole, created an atmosphere of safety and rightness that encouraged even the most reticent members to have their say. With each authentic expression, the inner world of the family gradually came to life, bringing tears, laughter and those elusive 'ah-ha' moments when truths are revealed and connected. However, what I noticed most was how the energy shifted from being stifled and shallow to being open and fluent, sometimes frenetic, sometimes serene, yet always respectful – Virginia wouldn't have it any other way. Intuitively I knew that what was taking place was real. At this level there is no place for platitudes or superficial strategies designed to satisfy external expectations. Here was the human family as I had never seen it before; Mamma, Papa and the kids without the trimmings, without the masks, and even more remarkably, without the fears. And it was wonderful - not only for those who participated, but also for those of us who had the privilege to just be there. As a professional I was there to watch a Master Therapist in action, but however much my mind tried to focus on the techniques of "Conjoint Family Therapy,' my heart was pulling in a different direction, reaching out to each member of the family and yearning for my own story to be told. This wasn't the Jacksons or the O'Malleys; it was my family - the Fewsters - struggling to be seen, to create connections, to become whole.

At the end of each session Virginia would ask the observers to share their thoughts and feelings, stressing the importance of making connection. Almost without exception, the feedback was personal and delivered with feeling. Watching members of the family take risks, expose their vulnerabilities and confront the barriers that stand between crisis and connection, we ended up being witnesses to ourselves. In this strange reversal, those who had done the work would listen intently to those who had watched, as one by one we brought ourselves into the arena. But there was a difference; we spoke alone and they listened as a family, connected and contained. I used to wonder how they could make this shift from such intense personal exchanges to dedicate their attention to the words of an outsider until it occurred to me that, much like individuals, families that are alive and aware on the inside are also able to set their own flexible boundaries.

As a therapist, I still wanted to know Virginia's secrets, to learn her techniques and replicate her forms, and I was not alone in this. No therapist has been more carefully watched and analyzed than Satir – even books have been written on the topic. Having seen many colleagues fail in their attempts to capture her magic, I came to the conclusion that the secret was more about the woman herself. For a few bizarre months I actually found myself trying to be like her, mouthing her words, imitating her gestures, expressing her attitudes and generally trying to assume her persona. Then it dawned on me that the real secret was for me to become more like Gerry Fewster, and as you are probably aware by now, that's a story in itself.

From Satir onwards, the idea of the family as a system became entrenched in the minds of theorists and practitioners alike. As the theories became more complex, the models more sophisticated and the techniques more intricate, my own enthusiasm began to wane. The 'system' was no longer the framework but the focus of the enterprise. Virginia's curiosity about and concern for individuals was replaced by a detached obsession with the model, and her impressive presence and interpersonal skills were distilled into repetitive communication techniques. Whenever I had the opportunity to watch the leading exponents in action, I invariably came away disheartened. With few exceptions, that wonderful opening up of energy generated through authentic expression was sadly missing. The basic stance was that once the family system could be identified, it could be influenced or modified through strategic forms of external intervention. At one point in my career, I came across a hospital based family therapy program in which the chief therapist, a psychiatrist, used video monitors to track six simultaneous sessions while communicating his observations and instructions to each individual therapist through microphone and a small receiving device clipped to the practitioner's left ear.

The Family as a 'Complex' System

It's not enough to say the family is a system and leave it at that. One of the many reasons why the new breed of family therapists stumbled in Satir's footsteps is that the system she used as a conceptual framework was not the same as theirs. Contemporary Systems Theory incorporates a vast multitude of models, and once again, I make no claim to being an expert. So in order to make my point I will settle for the most general propositions and the most obvious conclusions. Let me begin with the assumption that all relationships are 'systemic' whether we are talking about the behavior of sub-atomic particles, the evolution of the galaxies or the relationship between one adult and one child. From this broad perspective, all systems fall into one of two particular categories.

Simple systems are the stuff of Newtonian physics. They operate mechanically and predictably with each part playing a specified role in the functioning of the whole, much like a wind-up clock or a car engine. When they are working efficiently, simple systems are inherently repetitive and move toward a state of optimal balance, or homeostasis. Their efficiency can be enhanced through external manipulation – technological modifications or fine-tuning. Complex or emergent systems belong to the world of quantum physics. Within these configurations, each part possesses the ability to inform every other part through the expression of its own unique potential. In sharing this information, all parts operate together to form a collective and dynamic whole. As an emerging entity, the experience of the whole in turn, informs and influences the parts to produce a system that has its own specific purposes and its own internal integrity. Such systems, if they remain 'healthy,' are constantly moving toward increased growth and complexity. Theoretically, their potential is infinite. The key to growth is the availability of new and accurate information that can be accessed and assimilated by all parts and at all levels. Some of this information is generated internally and some is drawn from the outside, the broader context in which the system operates. Deficits or distortions from either source limit the developmental possibilities. All this implies that the system is 'intrinsically motivated,' seeking out new information in the service of its own purposes.

Both types of system rely upon the same universal force – energy. In general the simple system draws its energy from the outside. A clock works when wound up or energized by electricity, and a car engine runs on the energy stored within its fossil fuels. While all energy is drawn from a single source, complex systems are constantly generating their own energetic requirements through their internal activity. In both cases the system will fail to operate effectively if the flow of energy is disrupted or blocked, and will simply close down if the energy is withdrawn. By the same token, if the system is to maintain its overall purpose and internal unity, the energy of the parts and the whole must be contained within specific parameters or boundaries.

Understanding the essential difference between these two systemic arrangements is absolutely critical for anyone who wishes to examine any aspect of life, particularly human relations, from a systemic perspective. For example equating the human mind with the human brain and using the computer as an analogous model makes absolutely no sense. Yet psychology continues to rely on simple system models to develop its brands of theory and methodology. Not surprisingly the formulations remain mechanistic and the conclusions lifeless. But if we begin with the proposition that all systems involving human motivation and consciousness are potentially complex arrangements that, given the right conditions, are capable of infinite growth and development, the picture changes dramatically – remember Virginia Satir?

In human relations, the 'right' conditions are those in which each Self (a complex system in its own right) is free to express its potential within the experience of the whole. In order to play its part in the overall scheme, each individual Self must be connected to the whole yet have its own defined place – its own energetic and functional boundaries. Consciousness, or awareness, implies that the necessary external and internal information is communicated and assimilated effectively. This is referred to as an "open" system, one in which the parts and the whole operate from the same unrestricted informational base. Such an ideal may be difficult to imagine in the imperfect world of human relations, but that's not the point. The important issue is a matter of degree and whether the system in question is moving toward higher levels of openness and growth, or toward closure and atrophy. This can only be known through the subjective experience of the parts – the Selves directly involved in the system.

Viewed from this perspective, the human family offers an interesting case in point. A cynic might argue that the traditional family is essentially a closed system, more concerned with maintaining the distribution of power than the open sharing of information. To the degree that the family operates as a role-based arrangement, its members are restricted in their ability to express their own unique qualities and the energy becomes suppressed or blocked. Since such families are often locked into social and cultural

To the degree that the family operates as a role-based arrangement, its members are restricted in their ability to express their own unique qualities and the energy becomes suppressed or blocked.

prescriptions, information from the outside is strictly limited and systematically controlled. Under such conditions, the family may appear more like a simple mechanistic system, incapable of offering growth and development in whole or in part. Unfortunately this state of affairs is often the perspective assumed by behavioral scientists and celebrated in the name of family values.

While we all know families that operate this way (perhaps even our own), most of us are also aware of families that maintain high levels of openness and energy without sacrificing their inherent structure or purpose. Elders are respected, roles are acknowledged and children are cherished. Youngsters who grow up in such families are encouraged to bring themselves fully into the collective life of the family, each making his or her unique contribution to the whole. Everybody has a place that carries specific responsibilities, yet the system remains responsive to new information, and all members have the room to grow and the freedom to express themselves in their own way. Subjectively, each person lives within the family and the family lives within each person. Within the system personal boundaries are respected, and as part of the broader context, the family is contained and responsive to the outside world. Such families are never complete, ideal, or perfect. They are simply evolving personal environments in which new learning is an ever present and welcomed possibility – they are creative and complex systems.

So, have I managed to outline what such a family would look like and specified what we might do to make it work? On both counts, the answer is 'yes and no'.

Throughout this book I have talked about the development of the Self along its pathway toward authentic expression and relational autonomy. I have also stressed the need for us to rediscover our inherent relatedness to each other, to the planet we share and to the universe in which we all participate. Short of an apocalyptic disaster, it's probably safe to say that the family will retain its place as the primary context in which these things can be learned and experienced. If we move toward energizing this configuration from the inside out, there is no doubt that the family unit will change in both form and function. But if we try to shape its form or pre-determine its function, its natural evolution will grind to a halt. Even if we try to predict potential outcomes, the integrity of the process will be compromised. So what can we do? Well, we can always begin by exploring and sharing what 'is' and allowing what 'might be' to emerge from this place of connection.

Best Wishes from My Family to Yours

However we might conceptualize, or re-conceptualize the human family, this network of emotional bonds and genetic connections is one of nature's most exquisite designs. As with all species, its basic structure serves the function of survival, while its specific forms vary according to particular needs and circumstances. Given our unique ability to redefine our needs and modify our circumstances, we are able to create our own variations rather than drive around in the factory model. If we wish to preserve the integrity of the original, there is only so far we can go with our modifications. In this case we are dealing with our most profound human and developmental needs and creating a family is as close as we can come to co-creating with the natural order. If we part company here, why would we expect to find reconnection somewhere in the forests or out on the ocean? If this is to take place later in adulthood, it can only happen through conscious and dedicated remedial work. For this reason, I agree wholeheartedly with those who argue that the family and its associated values are central to our well being, if not our survival. My problem is that I usually find myself questioning the rigidity of their form and rejecting what they consider to be its essential values.

Being close to nature means experiencing our connection to our Selves and each Other. While the family of the future might not be the context for our closest and most intimate relationships, it will always be the point of origin for whatever we choose to create. A family that is consciously created and energetically connected invites its members to participate fully in life and serves as a microcosm for the whole. On the other hand, a family locked into some rigid prescription of roles and rituals, freezes consciousness, stifles creative energy and commits its members to repetitive and redundant ways of being. In this way it remains detached from, and unresponsive to, nature's purpose. Herein lay both the paradox and the irony. We are not apes or rabbits, and only by stepping out of the forms we have considered to be nature's decree will we play our part in the unfolding of the natural order – to bring consciousness and creativity into the cosmic equation. Nature has granted us this freedom to move within her realm and we can do no less than accept this incredible invitation. The paradox is that we are our creations and inextricably a part of that same realm. The irony is that our 'creativity' has become toxic to the territory and we appear to be on the brink of deportation. Like the second family described above, our beliefs have become rigid, our consciousness has become frozen and our ways of being have become shallow and repetitive. In our fear we may use our technological brilliance to create a patchwork of defensive measures but in nature's realm, there is only one possible solution – reconnection, or should I say, rapprochement.

If we have what it takes to move in this direction, I can think of no better focus than the future of our children. You may have more lofty concerns but for me, this provides a compelling reason to set about dismantling our illusions and pretensions, and confront the demons that continue to keep us fearful and apart. To some degree my stance is sentimental, but I like to believe it is also insightful, pragmatic and delightfully ironic. Wouldn't it be wonderful if our children became the resources through which we learned how to be in the world and with each other – our bridge to the next stretch along the developmental continuum?

EPILOGUE

So that's it. As I said at the outset, it was never my intention to convince you to change your mind about anything. All I asked was for you to take another look at childhood from your own experience and let the chips fall where they may. If you have stayed with me through the last seven chapters, I will consider my task accomplished. My beliefs are simply my beliefs, no more valid or enlightened than yours, and the evidence I have presented is indisputably selective and purposeful. Much as I might wish for others to share my concerns, my ambitions end at the point of being heard. Should you have any doubts about this, let me assure you that I reserve the right to modify or reverse anything I said, with or without notice. Meanwhile if I have masqueraded as an expert, you are free to judge me accordingly. Given a choice I would much rather be judged for my naivety than my pretenses.

The one truth I'd like to retain is my heartfelt commitment to the well being of children. Even this could be a sham; a disguised attempt to obtain insurance against the prospect of death and eternal damnation. The trouble is, no matter how much we pay the premiums by obeying the code or chasing enlightenment, the underlying anxiety is never far away. And so it will remain, until we come to recognize uncertainty as the essence of our freedom. By allowing ourselves the divine right to be wrong, we open up to infinite possibilities and purposes, not so much as discoverers but as creators. If this should turn out to be our role in the implicate order, it seems reasonable to expect that the central voice would speak back whenever our creations run contrary to the integrity of the whole, and we would be well advised to listen. But if we decide to cut ourselves off from the source through deafness, denial, confrontation or sheer arrogance, then we will have chosen to give up our place in the order – and should this come to pass, who's to say it is wrong?

Meanwhile all we can do is pass on whatever we have created to those who follow in our footsteps. For generations, we have been preparing our offspring to survive and compete in a world of winners and losers. Now we are beginning to realize that these values and aspirations are no longer sustainable, so what should we be teaching our children? If the majority of scientists are correct in their predictions, we could be wrestling with the core issues of physical survival well within the lifespan of the current generation. How many of us has anything useful to contribute to such a desperate cause? Yet if we remain on our present heading, the prospects are bleak indeed; the most likely scenario being a vicious scramble for the last of the planet's resources until even the fittest find themselves struggling to survive. If there are survivors, I wonder who these resilient Souls might be? Will they be those dedicated to the creation of conscious and sustainable communities, or are they more likely to be the scavengers living by their wits and destroying whatever appears to stand in their way?

If I were a man of science, I might tell you how we have moved too far along the evolutionary trail to return to the raw savagery of our ancestors. If I were a religious man, I might invite you to join in my prayers for divine intervention and sweet salvation. But then, I am neither and whatever faith I have lies elsewhere. Based upon this faith, I have chosen to believe that the human Spirit is an indestructible and incorruptible element within the cosmos, and every expression of that Spirit is a step toward wholeness. Such steps are not taken on the stairway to the stars, but through the unexplored alleyways that lie between one human being and another. Whatever the future holds, I am firmly convinced that until we are prepared to make a conscious and determined shift in this direction, our place on the planet will continue to be tenuous. I can think of no better way of rising to this challenge than by taking the first critical steps toward those who need us most - the children in our care. This may not prevent the apocalypse many are predicting, but within the broader scheme, the reconnection of one Spirit to an Other can only serve the universal cause – an affirmation of our place in the scheme of things.

I have no idea whether this offers any hope for our troubled world, but hope can be a hollow illusion – an imaginary escape from what 'is' to dream up some fantasy around what 'should be.' The human Spirit is undoubtedly a powerful force and the extent of our creative abilities remains unknown; but the hubris that leads us to believe we can continue to manipulate nature into serving our adolescent fantasies is probing to be a fatal delusion. Wherever we choose to look, the evidence of our alienation from the natural order is painfully apparent. How many warnings do we need before we come to accept the certainty of uncertainty and learn how to explore and respond within a system that is infinitely greater than the sum of its parts? What will it take for us to reject the assurances of the power brokers and begin to create the conditions in which the Spirit can thrive in its human form on a planet that has always offered this opportunity?

These are questions that call for the highest levels of individual awareness and can only be resolved through collective commitment. If you believe there's an easier way, take a look at the leaders we have allowed or assigned, to tackle the issues that now threaten our species. Do these people personify the highest levels of human consciousness, compassion and integrity? Are these people you would trust to act in your best interests when their own ambitions are on the line? And what about their solutions? Are their designs intended to promote the health of the planet and the well being of humanity as a whole? Do their actions reflect a deep and enduring concern for those who already hover on the edge of survival?

If you have answered most of these questions in the affirmative, I have nothing further to add. But if your responses are less than positive, you may wish to ask yourself why these particular people are calling the shots and what the central voice might have to say about their intentions? Just imagine you are that central voice, and while you might not feel personally empowered to change the world, the roots of the problem could well be embedded in your silence and complicity. The best way to hear that voice is to speak it, and should you find yourself listening to the truth, the only way to make it known is to share it. And should you feel so inclined, might I suggest that you whisper it into the ears of those who most desperately need to hear – the children. In the moment of divine revelation, it may turn out to be erroneous, but it would almost certainly be an improvement on what they're getting now. In the long run, we may even generate the support I'm seeking for my most basic and enduring proposition – by connecting with ourselves through our relationships with our children, we will grow together, and together we can change the world.

BIBLIOGRAPHY

Ainsworth, M. (1972). *Attachment and dependency: A comparison.* In J. Ferwirtz (Ed.), Attachment and dependency. Cambridge, England: Cambridge University Press.

Balint, M. (1968). *The Basic Fault.* London: Tavistock.

Bettelheim, B. (1987). *A Good Enough Parent.* New York: Alfred A. Knopf.

Bohm, D. (1980). *Wholeness and the Implicate Order*, London: Routledge & Keegan Paul.

Bowlby, J. (1969). *Attachment and Loss: Vol. 1. Attachment.* New York: Basic Books.

Bowlby, J. (1973). *Attachment and Loss: Vol. 2. Separation, anxiety, and anger.* New York: Basic Books.

Bradley, R. A. (1996). *Husband-Coached Childbirth.* New York: Bantam Books.

Brenner, P. (1981). *Life is a Shared Creation.* Marina del Rey, CA: DeVorss & Co.

Caldwell, C. (Ed.) (1997). *Getting in Touch: The Guide to the New Body-Centered Therapies.* Wheaton, IL: Quest Books.

Chilton Pearce, J. (1992). *Evolution's End: Claiming the Potential of Our Intelligence.* San Francisco: Harper Collins.

(a) Chamberlain, D. (1999). *Selected Works by David Chamberlain. Special Millennium Issue, Journal of Prenatal and Perinatal Psychology & Health 14 (1-2).*

(b) Chamberlain, D. (1994). *How pre- and perinatal psychology can transform the world. Pre- and Perinatal Psychology Journal 8(3).*

Cline, F. (1992). *Hope for High Risk and Rage Filled Children.* Evergreen, CO: E.C. Publications.

Danesi, M. (1998). *Cool: The Signs and Meanings of Adolescence.* University of Toronto Press.

Deci, E. (1975). *Intrinsic Motivation.* New York: Plenum Press.

Emerson, W. (1977). *Birth Trauma: The Psychological Effects of Obstetrical Interventions.* Petaluma, Ca: Emerson Training Seminars.

Fowles, J. (1968). *The Aristos.* London: Pan Books.

Gatto, J.T. (1992). *Dumbing Us Down.* Philadelphia, PA: New Society Publishers

Gleick, J. (1988). *Chaos: Making a New Science.* New York: Penguin

Glasser, W. (1969). *Schools Without Failure.* New York: Harper & Row.

Helmstetter, S. (1989). *Choices.* New York: Pocket Books.

Holt, J. (1964). *How Children Fail.* New York: Pitman Publishing Co.

Iacoboni, M. (2008) *Mirroring People.* New York: Picador

Jaynes, J. (1976). *The Origins of Consciousness in the Breakdown of the Bicameral Mind.* Boston, MA: Houghton Mifflin.

Janov, A. (1970). *The Primal Scream.* New York: Dell Publishing Co.

Kohl, H. *The Open Classroom: A Practical Guide to a New Way of Teaching*. New York: Random House.

Laing, R.D. (1976). *The Facts of Life*. London: Penguin Books.

Leboyer, F. (1975). *Birth Without Violence*. New York: Alfred Knopf.

Lieberman, M. (1970). *Smoking and the Fetus*. American Journal of Obstetrics, August 5.

Leonard, G. (1968). *Education and Ecstasy*. Berkeley, CA: North Atlantic Books.

Liedloff, J. (1975). *The Continuum Concept*. New York: Addison-Wesley Publishing Company, Inc.

Lipton, B. (2005). *The Biology of Belief*. Santa Rosa, CA: Mountain of Love/Elite Books.

Louv, R. (2006). *Last Child in the Woods*. Chapel Hill, NC: Algonquin Books.

Miller, A. (1981). *Prisoners of Childhood*. New York: Basic Books.

Mitford, J. (1992). *The American Way of Birth*. New York: Dutton.

Morris, D. (1969). *The Naked Ape*. London: Jonathon Cape.

Neill, A.S. (1960). *Summerhill: A Radical Approach to Child Rearing*. New York: Hart Publishing.

Odent, M. (2006). *The Long Term Consequences of How We Are Born. Journal of Prenatal and Perinatal Psychology and Health 21(2)*.

Paris, T. & Paris, E. (1992). *I'll Never Do to My Kids What My Parents Did to Me*. Los Angeles: Lowell House.

Pert, C. (1997). *Molecules of Emotion*. New York: Touchstone.

Polanyi, M. (1958) *Personal Knowledge: Toward a Post-Critical Philosophy*

Rank, O. (1929). *The Trauma of Birth*. New York: Harcourt Brace.

Reich, W. (1961). *Character Analysis*. New York: Farrar, Strauss & Giroux.

Rosenberg, J., Rand, M. and Asay, D. (1985). *Body, Self and Soul: Sustaining Integration*. Atlanta: Harmonics

Rosenberg, J., and Kitaen-Morse, B. (1996). *The Intimate Couple*. Atlanta: Turner Publishing.

Schutz, W. (1984). *The Truth Option*. Berkeley, CA: Ten Speed Press.

Silberman, C.E. (1970). *Crisis in the Classroom*. New York: Random House.

Siegal, D.J. and Hartzell, M. (2004). *Parenting from the Inside Out*. New York: Tarcher/Penguin.

Sonne, J.C. (2000). *Abortion Survivors At Columbine*. Journal of Prenatal and Perinatal Psychology and Health. 15 (1).

Stanley, L. (1994). *Unassisted Childhood*. New York: Greenwood Publishing Group.

Stern, D. (1985). *The Interpersonal World of the Infant*. New York: Basic Books.

Verny, T. with Kelly, J. (1981). *The Secret Life of the Unborn Child*. Toronto: Collins.

Wilber, K. (1977). *The Spectrum of Consciousness*. Wheaton, Ill: Quest.

Winnicot, D.W. (1996). *Thinking About Children*. Reading, MA: Addison-Wesley.

Wong, B. and McKeen, J. (1998). *The New Manual for Life*. Gabriola: P.D. Publishing.

Zohar, D. (1990). *The Quantum Self*. New York: William Morrow and Company Inc.

Appendix A

Breath as the Gateway to the Self

Throughout this book, I invited you to consider the core Self as a felt sense of well being in the body and that the most natural and effective means of access is through the breath.

When we breathe slowly and deeply, we relax and become open to our feelings. Conversely, if our breathing is rapid and shallow we tighten up, diverting energy away from our feelings in order to increase our state of physical and mental alertness. For the most part this all takes place beyond our awareness and is regulated by the autonomic nervous system (ANS). Centered in the more primitive regions of the brain, the functions of the ANS are essentially 'involuntary' and our individual responses reflect the history of our dealings with the outside world. If our experiences have been predominantly stressful, our natural breathing patterns will tend to be rigid and our feelings repressed. Alternatively if our encounters with the world have been generally assuring and stress-free, our breathing will be full and our feelings accessible. As with most of our learning the basic patterns are established very early in life.

Along with respiration, the ANS also controls the organs and emotions through the endocrine system. Simply stated this system has two components – the 'sympathetic' and the 'parasympathetic.' The sympathetic mode, often identified as the 'freeze, fight or flight' response, prepares us for action by increasing heart and respiration rates along with the flow of adrenalin. The parasympathetic works in the opposite direction, slowing down heart and respiration rates to support a state of relaxation in which emotions and feelings can be fully experienced. In any given situation, the 'triggering' of sympathetic or parasympathetic responses depends upon whether we perceive the external conditions to be hostile and threatening, or friendly and supportive.

Unlike other creatures we are able to override and re-program the ANS by intentionally modifying our perceptions, creating new meanings and constructing our own realities. We can also engage its functions directly through various breathing techniques. By consciously breathing deeply into our bellies, we can purposefully create a state of relaxation: alternatively, by bringing our breath into the upper chest, we can increase the level of energy in our bodies. When we combine these two processes, we can build and release the energetic flow in our bodies to enhance our feelings of aliveness and well being. These are the conditions in which the core Self can become experienced directly and expressed. It should be pointed out that these conscious interventions will not ensure ongoing access to internal experience; this will occur only when through regular practice, such changes become incorporated into the natural unconscious breathing patterns.

Exercise One: Opening the Body

Find a quiet and comfortable place where you can lie down with your knees up and your feet making solid contact with the floor. This makes it possible for you to 'ground,' rather than discharge, your energy. Alternatively you may prefer to sit in a comfortable chair, again with your feet firmly planted.

Once you are settled close your eyes and take your awareness into your body. Notice how easy or difficult it is to make this shift. Become aware of how your body feels in general – open or closed, light or heavy, tight or relaxed etc. Pay particular attention to specific sensations and where they are located in your body – warmth, cold, numbness, aches and pains etc. Be aware of how it feels to be in your body – comfortable or uncomfortable, familiar or unfamiliar. Notice your breathing – deep or shallow, fast or slow, easy or strained, rhythmic or jerky. Resist any temptation to make adjustments; your concern is with what 'is,' rather than what 'should be'. Don't rush; your body will need time to find its voice and respond to your inquiry. Listen carefully as a curious internal witness. If you find yourself moving back into your head, gently allow any thoughts to pass and take your awareness back into your body on the exhale.

When you feel a sense of connection with your body and breath, open your eyes and begin by taking four or five deep belly breaths through your mouth with your throat open. The emphasis should be on a long *unforced* out-breath. It might help to make a sound, such as a sigh, as the breath leaves your body. You may also wish to place a hand over your navel to feel a comforting sense of contact, applying a slight pressure on the out-breath. After five or six breaths, close your eyes, take your awareness back into your body and notice whatever you notice. Does your body feel different in any way? If so, how and where? If you experience particular feelings or emotions allow your breath to explore and express them without restriction.

By repeating this procedure several times, your body will begin to open up, offering more varied and detailed information. All you need to do is acknowledge this communication and notice where in your body the feelings and sensations are located. Above all, avoid any temptation to intervene in whatever is happening – this is all about *awareness* and there's nothing that needs to be fixed or changed.

Exercise Two: Building an Energy Charge

Once you sense your body is open and responsive, you can increase the flow of information by drawing more energy into the system. This is accomplished by bringing your breath into the upper chest using a technique known as 'charge breathing.' Here the object is to expand the rib cage from the top down.

To bring attention to this area, gently press your thumbs or index fingers into two acupressure points located just under the clavicle and directly above the nipples. With a little exploration you will recognize these points as small indentations that may be tender or sensitive to touch. By bringing your breath to meet these points, you will know if your upper chest is actually expanding and not simply moving up and down. Another check is to make sure your shoulders are remaining level. In charge breathing the emphasis is on the inhalation with the exhalation being allowed to fall out naturally without effort.

With your eyes, mouth and throat open, take five or six charge breaths into your upper chest. Close your eyes and focus your attention to the inside, allow the energy to spread and track its movement through your body. Notice where it flows easily and where it seems to become sticky or blocked. Be aware of any new or any sensations like tingling, openness, numbness or changes in temperature. . If you find yourself becoming lightheaded or dizzy, slow down and allow your body to resumed its own natural rhythm. After a minute or so, open your eyes and repeat the exercise with five or six more charge breaths.

Charge breathing should be practiced slowly and gently until your body adjusts to taking in more breath and energy. With this you may experience a rush of energy along with intensified sensations or emotions. As always the key is to stay with whatever is happening. But remember, a body that has been protecting for years is unlikely to reveal its secrets at the first invitation – be gentle and patient. All breathing involves the diaphragm and like any other muscle, this structure that stretches across the rib cage, needs graduated exercise to develop its strength and flexibility. When the diaphragm moves freely, it descends just beneath the lower ribs on the in-breath and ascends up toward the sternum on the out-breath. This movement promotes the fullness of the breathing cycle – inhale and exhale in a seamless sequence – and ensures the unrestricted flow of energy through the body.

Living with varying degrees of stress or anxiety, as most of us do, we develop characteristic ways of restricting the movement of the diaphragm, thereby interrupting the flow of energy. Over time, these restrictive breathing practices show up as holding patterns in the musculature that profoundly influence our physical, emotional and psychological well being. Charge breathing brings us up against these energetic blocks, and if we move too quickly or intensively, we run the risk of strengthening their resistance. The object of the exercise is to let go of the old restrictive breathing patterns by allowing the body to relax and release the energetic blocks gently and incrementally. In order to consciously enhance your breathing efficiency, you must also begin to let go of the old restrictive breathing patterns you have unconsciously constructed over the years.

The Full Breath to the Self

With practice, you will be able to increase the flow of energy in your body even more effectively by shuttling back and forth between charge breathing and release breathing. The overall subjective experience is one of increased aliveness, along with a deeper sense of health and well being. After practicing the breathing exercises, take the time to go inside and breathe normally. Over time, you will notice how your natural breathing patterns change to a deeper and fuller rhythm. From the inside, you will become aware of a growing sense of well being that seems pulsate from a particular location in your body. Focus on that place and allow your breath to explore and express it fully. This is the essence of Self-awareness, the center of your knowing and your birthright as a conscious, unique and connected human being.

APPENDIX B

Exchanging Mirrors

Accurate mirroring makes it possible for us to be seen and heard by another person – not only for how we appear on the outside but also for our experiences on the inside. This enables the Self to become recognized, known and expressed in our closest relationships. Our ability to offer an accurate mirror to an Other, is directly related to how well we have been mirrored, particularly during early childhood when the Self is seeking to establish its place in the world. Although very few of us received on-going accurate mirroring during this phase of development, it is possible to make up for any deficiencies later in life through awareness and practice. We developed the exercise "Exchanging Mirrors" for our work with couples but, any two people who wish to experience being mirrored and enhance their own mirroring skills can use the following procedures.

Setting the scene

Sit face-to-face at a distance that feels comfortable for both. If you take a deep breath and notice the feelings or sensations, your body will tell you whether you are too close or distant. Try various distances until you <u>both</u> feel comfortable. This is called establishing a 'contact boundary.'

Using yarn, string or chalk, make a circle around yourself that delineates your personal space. Take a full breath and imagine yourself filling that space. If it feels too large or too small change it accordingly. Then ask your partner to create a personal boundary in the same way.

Having a boundary means that all your perceptions, thoughts and feelings, even about the other person, belong to you and not to them. All you can share is your own experience. This stance might create some confusion at first but it is essential for both offering and accepting a mirror. When offering mirroring feedback, you might begin by saying, "This is all about me, and not about you," until this idea is fully accepted and understood. The boundary lets you know where one person ends and the other begins

Level One

The first glimpses – reflective listening

First decide who will speak first (A) and who will mirror (B).

'A' begins by sharing whatever feelings they have in the moment - excitement, anxiety, embarrassment etc. B listens, paying attention to both the words and the feeling content behind them. At this stage, not all feelings need to be disclosed, but whatever is shared must be real and honestly expressed.

B responds by stating *in their own words* what they have heard and what they understand about A's experience. Simply repeating the other person's words stifles the process – people need a responsive mirror, not a stuffed parrot.

B then asks A to comment on the accuracy of their understanding. A can clarify, modify or elaborate while B simply listens without responding.

Before changing over, A and B close their eyes, take a breath and reflect upon the exchange, while paying particular attention to their own feelings. Taking time to check in with the Self is a good habit to establish at this stage.

Roles are reversed as B shares their feelings in the moment and A responds by offering a mirror. Bear in mind that B now has much more information to work with. After the feedback, B has the opportunity to clarify, modify or elaborate upon A's understanding.

This back-and-forth procedure may be repeated several times in the course of the first session. Over time the process becomes more conversational with each person deciding what they want to say. As long as there is honesty on both sides, the mirroring practice can continue regardless of the conversational content.

Before closing the session, each shares what they have learned about the other and ask for accuracy feedback. Each person then reveals the degree to which they have felt seen and heard by the other.

Level Two

Looking deeper – energetic resonance and attunement

With practice, each person's mirroring will become more accurate and validated. The key ingredients are: (a) unfettered curiosity; (b) honesty; (c) personal presence for Self and Other, (d) trusting feelings and intuition. The skill to be developed is called 'reflective listening." When both parties feel competent at this level, it's time to move to the deeper level – energetic resonance and attunement. Here we are concerned with creating the energetic contact beyond thoughts and words. The essential understanding is that we can only respond to another person's feelings by experiencing and expressing our own. Energetic mirroring connects one core Self to an Other and facilitates the development of 'accurate empathy.'

At this level it is important that the boundary procedures outlined above are followed before each session. These boundaries can be re-adjusted at any time throughout at the request of either person. A mirror that is either too close or too far away will be either distorted or vague.

B begins by inviting A to talk about a time in their lives when they felt particularly happy – an event or circumstances. Beyond listening to the words, B's primary task is to become aware of their own internal experience and incorporate this into the mirror. The appropriate stance is not, " I know how *you* feel" but "I know how *I* feel – does this relate to your experience?" Now the mirror not only reflects the words, but also the feelings behind them. As before, A is asked to provide accuracy feedback.

When this is complete, A asks B to talk about a time when *they* were happy and the same procedure is followed. In concluding this first exchange it is a good idea to take a few minutes to 'debrief' by simply reviewing what has taken place.

B then invites A to talk about a time when they felt particularly sad and the cycle is repeated. This process may be extended to include a range of emotions, including anger, frustration, fear, confusion etc.

At the conclusion, both parties have the opportunity to share what they have learned about themselves and each other through the session.

With practice, the above procedures will make it possible for both individuals to become more accurately tuned-in to their own and each other's internal experiences. The energetic-feeling level is just a complex as the verbal cognitive level and any single event may entail a range of differentiated feelings and responses. The next step offers an opportunity to explore this domain a little further by fine-tuning understanding and mirroring skills.

B begins by asking A to talk about their life over the past year – the highs, the lows, the hopes, the fears etc. Rather than wait for the entire story to unfold, B offers a mirror at various points along the way. Choosing the right moment to intervene is a critical aspect of mirroring to be learned and practiced. The skill is the ability to invite reflections without interrupting the flow of the story. The quality and timing of these interventions should be incorporated into A's feedback before the roles are reversed.

Exploration at this level can be continued through reciprocal sharing and mirroring on topics of particular interest to one or both individuals. These may include specific events, thoughts about the past, present or future, hopes, wishes and aspirations, etc. etc. For committed individuals, this can also include whatever is current within their personal or professional relationship.

Effective energetic mirroring is not only about a congruence of particular feeling states, it also involves matching the energy level of the Other. If the energy level of mirroring person is significantly greater or less than that of the Other, the connection will be proportionately compromised. Learning to attune energetically is an integral part of the process that can be assisted by honest and accurate feedback from the receiver.

Level Three

Seeing the world through the eyes of an Other – perspective and role taking ability

The following exercise will be useful to those who wish to better understand the world in which the other person lives. It can be conducted in a familiar setting such as a home or office, or wherever the two people can be together without external distractions.

Person A sits immediately behind B, as close as their boundaries will allow but without physically touching. Couples in a close or intimate relationship often find it more comfortable to sit on the floor with A's legs stretched out on either side of B's hips. Whatever position is chosen, the idea is that A is able to look out from behind B's head at the same eye level.

Once comfortable, B looks around the room and reports whatever draws their attention. Once this initial orientation is complete, B picks out objects that have particular meaning or relevance – this may because of their familiarity or they may trigger thoughts and memories of other places and/or experiences. This is an exercise in 'free association' – whatever comes to mind is immediately shared without explanation. A clock, for example, may remind the person of a clock in grandmother's kitchen, or it may be a symbol of B's lifelong stance of 'so much to do and so little time.' Either perception may trigger an emotional thought or memory that may, or may not, be expressed. This may not move easily at first but as the person becomes at ease with the process it usually turns out to be a fascinating revelation of how much we respond to the world based upon our experiences of the past. A remains silent throughout.

After A and B have exchanged roles each can reflect upon their experience through the exercise while the other intervenes at appropriate times to offer a verbal and energetic mirror – more practice.

The Self in the looking glass

As you move through any or all of the above exercises, whatever thoughts and feelings you have become grist for the mill and with a little courage and perseverance, can be incorporated into the mirroring process. As you and your partner become increasingly attuned, the revelations and understandings become progressively deeper and the interaction becomes freer flowing. People who have traveled this road invariably report a new level of closeness and are frequently amazed by what they discover about themselves, each other and their relationship.

Mirroring children

All children need to be mirrored for who they really are. For this to occur the adult must remain fully present in his or her own personal boundary and have no agenda other than to respond honestly to child's experience. This might begin with 'reflective listening' – paraphrasing (not simply repeating) what the child says. At the deeper level, the essential stance of the adult is curiosity and authentic responsiveness to the youngster's feelings – to match sadness with sadness and joy with joy. There should be no expectation of equal reciprocity as the young Self is still seeking a place in the world. On the other hand, children are naturally curious and those who have been mirrored in this way will move on to create reciprocal and empathic relationships as the Self becomes increasingly expressed and known.

INDEX

FURTHER INFORMATION

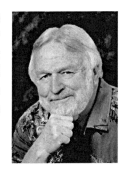

Gerry Fewster is President of the Serenity Child and Parent Society Board of Directors, Administrator of the Pacific North West IBP Institute and Associate Adjunct Professor in the Department of Applied Psychology at the University of Calgary.

For information on workshops, trainings and consultations offered by Gerry and Judith Fewster please contact...
www.DontLetYourKidsBeNormal.com

LaVergne, TN USA
10 November 2010
204200LV00004B/16/P